The What When Wine Diet

Paleo and Intermittent Fasting for Health and Weight Loss

by Melanie Avalon

Jerry,

Thank you so much for welcoming me into the Fleming's family! I am so grateful, and truly loving it. I look forward to many moments and memories to come! You definitly foster an incredible atmosphere in the restaurant. I also wish you the Merriest of Christmases, and an epic New Year!

Warmest,
Melanie

P.S- I love all your wine + movie trivia!

© 2015 Melanie Avalon

All rights reserved. No part of this publication may be reproduced, distributed, or transmitted in any form or by any means, including photocopying, recording, or other electronic or mechanical methods, without the prior written permission of the publisher, except in the case of brief quotations embodied in critical reviews and certain other noncommercial uses permitted by copyright law.

Published in Los Angeles, California by *Incandescent Expressions*.

Note To Readers: *The What When Wine Diet* is composed of personal experiences, ideas, and research. It is not providing professional medical service, and is not intended to replace the care of a physician. The author and publisher are in no way responsible for any liability or loss which may occur from the contents of this book… including weight loss of course.

All referenced products, restaurants, menus, etc. are subject to change. Any such mentions are of a personal opinion, and the author harbors no affiliation with such entities.

Cover Photo by Carmen Emmi.

ISBN-13: 978-0692458600

ISBN-10: 0692458603

DEDICATION

To my parents, for their eternal support in life. Thanks for providing the ingredients, so I could bake the proverbial (gluten-free) cake. Love you more, most, so much!

TABLE OF CONTENTS

Introduction	1
My Diet History	5
In Consideration of Calories	11

PART I: WHAT?

What is Paleo?	21
Grainy Problems	27
Sweet Problems	41
Fake Problems	51
Fat Problems	57
How To Do Paleo	69
Transitioning To Paleo	77
Shopping, Paleo Style	85
Dining, Paleo Style	93
Paleo Adherence Tips	103
Paleo Q&A	109

PART II: WHEN?

What Is Intermittent Fasting?	123
How To Do Intermittent Fasting	129
Tips For Intermittent Fasting	133
Intermittent Fasting Benefits	137
Why Intermittent Fasting Is Easy	145
The Myths of Metabolism	151
Fat Burning, IF Style	159
Exercise, IF Style	167
Intermittent Fasting Q&A	173

PART III: WINE?
    Alcohol and Diet   181

PART IV: AND?
    "Functional" Exercise   189
    #Dealing With Diet Backlash   199
    Supplements   203

Conclusion   217
Thanks   219
About The Author   221
Resources   223

INTRODUCTION

"Oh, are you picking out a steak?"

We were standing in line at the meat counter, not (as you might imagine) in some expensive health market proclaiming natural goodness, but rather in a mainstream grocery store on Sunset Boulevard, a street as glamorous as it is grimy. He surveyed my figure, proud of his clever quip, as though such carnivorous activity was obviously the last thing I was doing. I felt a smile shyly illuminate my face.

That was *exactly* what I was doing.

Growing up, I always strove for that "ideal" female body. I subscribed to the myriad of fat-burning *lose-10-pounds-in-10-days* promises saturating society, the perpetual magazine covers with auspiciously colorful letters. I bought into the ever new recycled fad, thinking perhaps *this* time I'd find some revolutionary tidbit of information not mentioned in the vast graveyard of similar claims, where tombstones bared epitaphs of *"he ran more"* and *"she ate less."*

Yet regardless of how much I exercised or how many calories I did (or did not) consume, my body stubbornly hovered at a basic weight it apparently deemed just dandy. And despite hours of cardio (25 mile bike rides on breezy summer days) and sincere efforts of ab exercises (300 crunches while watching *American Idol*), my composition simply didn't change that much. I never questioned the lack of progress. I just figured *I wasn't doing enough*.

While never "overweight" by official BMI standards, I

nevertheless desired a body instilling instant pride, rather than one I was constantly trying to perfect. What was it like to prance around in a bikini, without a single bodily care? I also assumed this glorious archetype would be restlessly hungry and difficult to possess, like slippery soap in a bathtub. I'd be bound to miserable exercise and diet restriction to keep it... but all would be worth it!

Beyond the common desire to lose weight, I also struggled with "normal" ailments attributed to the throes of existence: acne, blood sugar swings, lower back pain, and headaches. People say these are just a part of life, and I agreed. I never thought it might relate to food.

Then one day I auditioned a new diet protocol focused on *what* you eat rather than *how much* you eat. It was revolutionary. The thought of not considering calories was *absurd*. But the more I researched, the more I realized there was a *science* to diet. Common wisdom of calories and cardio carelessly dismissed the importance of hormonally encouraging the body to burn fat on a cellular level. Further research next led me to another complementary dietary outfit: this one focused on *when* you eat. (Hint: It's not all the time.) This also flew in the face of everything I'd been told in the 2 decades or so of my life.

My ever evolving obsession with nutritional science yielded not only a lower body weight, but a paradigm shift. Gone were the days of calorie counting and restriction, the yearning moments of sugary lust and scolding atonement. Years of self-experimentation led to the point where I am now unyoked from constant "dieting." Free from cravings and hunger. I eat delicious food to satiety without calorie counting, partake in minimal "exercise" by common standards, and yet am perfectly content with my thin, toned body. Oh, and my health has improved to boot!

I wrote this book to address the constant questions I get about my diet. I wanted to lay out everything I do, and why it works. Before embarking on this crazy writing adventure, I simply had my own "N of 1" experience to validate my claims of Paleo and intermittent fasting, supported by my obsessive engagement with the many related blogs and podcasts. For this book, however, I resolved to put my college degree to good use, and actually *research* everything. I was shocked by the findings: it was almost *too* easy. The amount of studies and trials validating the health benefits of low carb, Paleo, fasting, and even wine, is overwhelming. Please somebody tell me: how is this stuff *not* more mainstream already?

And lastly, a confession. I'm using weight loss as the lure for something better. If you start implementing the dietary changes and patterns I discuss, you will not only lose weight without restriction and cravings, but possibly experience a new side of health you didn't know existed! That being said, this book is my personal story, and I am ultimately libertarian in my approach to diet. I firmly believe in self-experimentation and finding what works *for you*. Maybe just Paleo will be your thing, or maybe just intermittent fasting will appeal. Try things and see what happens! You can do all of it, or pick and choose what you like. Everyone has his or her own beautiful path to follow in this crazy diet wonderland.

Really, what do you have to lose, except excess weight and its discontents?

My Diet History

I was not always as I am. (Are we ever?) My wanderings through diet wonderland encountered their fair share of neurotic tangents and self-experimentation, ultimately leading to where I am today: a happy, Paleo, intermittent faster sipping on a glass of Pinot Noir. While I continue to research and tweak things, I like to think I've reached a stable, sustainable diet lifestyle. Gone are the days of unfulfilling fads and phases. Let's take a walk down memory lane!

THE ADOLESCENT YEARS
 I grew up in the South consuming the typical Standard American Diet, with a particular fancy for starchy carbs and sugar. My ideal meal at such times would have featured Fettuccine Alfredo and Coca-Cola, with Funfetti cake for dessert. Sugar and flour were *yum yum delicious!* I liked my meat slathered in sauces, while vegetables were bland and boring. I'd eat the minimal amount of greens as insisted by my mother, then move on without a moment of regret. I disdained salads, *never* eating them. I did, however, silently envy those who *liked* salads. How fortunate for them.
 Despite my SAD diet (quite a telling acronym), I maintained a healthy weight on the thin side of normal, for which I thank good genes and the activity of youth. At age 15, however, I began birth control for acne, a skin condition plaguing me with *constant* embarrassment. While my skin did clear up a bit from the pill, I gained about 10 pounds, a substantial amount of weight relative to my body size, and an association I did not connect to the hormonal effects of the pill. After being accepted into the early entrance program at the University of Southern California the next year (It's

been real Memphis!), I dieted down a few pounds via calorie restriction, in sparkling anticipation of the horizon's alluring collegiate life.

My freshman year of college at USC conjured a whirlwind of buffet comfort foods and study nights fueled by ice cream and cookies. Who knows how many divine muffins I consumed from the resident "Trojan Grounds" coffee shop during that smashingly scholastic time. When I went on spring break that year with my family, I stepped on the hotel scale out of curiosity. To my chagrin, the number was 15 pounds more than when I started college. Oops. When did that happen?

Sophomore year of college, I decided to crack down and get back to my "high school self." Although a murderous route to follow, meticulous calorie counting became a consistent theme. I also tried anything and everything that looked promising, all with the goal of a certain scale number.

And I mean everything.

Cascading bottles of "promising" appetite suppressants, fat burning pills, and thermogenics filled my drawers. When I received an email saying one of my recently purchased "magic diet pills" was recalled, I proclaimed *"THIS STUFF MUST WORK!"* and guarded my bottle like a secret drug, saving it for "special occasions." It still lies in my supplement graveyard. I tried a semester of "Dr. Siegal's Cookie Diet," receiving massive shipments of "healthy" meal replacement cookies. I flirted with vegetarianism. (That didn't last long.) I made a foray into the HCG diet world. Nothing like sneaky clockwork bathroom trips to sublingually administer crystal liquid drops from a dark bottle to make you feel suspicious!

Then one day I stumbled upon a concept which would welcome a new era, changing my dietary escapades forever.

STAGE ONE: LOW CARB (c. Fall 2010)

On one unassuming evening of midterm procrastination, I found myself in the online "low carb" community, spearheaded (for better or worse) by the Atkins diet. Who knows how I got there. Before this point, all I remembered about Atkins was a high school friend saying the diet protocol was stupid, since she could eat a steak and not a carrot. Yep. That sounded pretty stupid.

Discovering the "scientific" aspect of a low carb diet, however, fascinated me. I was intrigued by the concept of "ketosis" - a metabolic state in which the body switches its primary fuel source from carbs (i.e.: sugar) to fat, generating "ketones" to supplement energy. I was thrilled that I could measure the presence of ketones in my body (and thus "measure" my fat loss in a sense) with urine reagent test strips. The first time the sample strip turned dark pink (signifying the presence of ketones), I leapt for joy. I called my mother, proclaiming, *"It's so scientific! I can literally measure my fat loss!"* She laughed at my enthusiasm. (Had she known the obsession which would eventually come from this finding, she may have reacted differently.)

Fascinated by the science of the diet, I began furiously plowing through low carb literature. The research seemed solid, and I was beginning to reap the physical benefits of the protocol. Along with weight loss, I began experiencing other beneficial changes: my energy levels, sleep, and skin all improved. As my body became "fat adapted," I no longer suffered blood sugar crashes. My body seemed to handle itself much better between meals. Gone were the feelings of a persistently unsatisfied appetite. I simply felt *different* as a person.

Maybe there was something to all this "health stuff?" Before low carb, I was the girl who loved tailored topical treatment. I saw all ailments of the body as unrelated and case specific. In no way was *diet* related to anything besides weight gain or weight loss. Internal supplements or diet changes for external conditions seemed unnecessarily slow and silly. Yet my adoption of a low carb way of eating was causing me to reevaluate the situation. I was beginning to think that perhaps what we put IN our bodies ultimately creates the foundation for our state of health, holistically affecting everything.

STAGE TWO: INTERMITTENT FASTING (c. Spring 2011)

Going low carb was a healthy and beneficial step in my diet history, but calorie counting slyly became replaced with carb counting. I began fixating on the exact carb count of each morsel I ingested, worrying about superseding my maximum number of grams per day, and thus getting "kicked out" of ketosis. One neuroses replaced another.

Then one day I stumbled upon Rusty Moore's online blog post, "Lose Body Fat By Eating Just One Meal Per Day?" Detailing the concept of "Intermittent Fasting," Moore suggested that eating all of your food in a concentrated time window of a few hours, rather than spread throughout the day, would not only encourage weight loss, but boost one's health in general. Hundreds of reader comments and testimonials lauded the benefits.

This idea flew in the face of *everything* I'd been told about dieting. Skipping meals was terrible for the body! Didn't I need to eat constantly to keep my metabolism going? However, as I was becoming increasingly suspicious of popular diet wisdom, was never much of a breakfast person anyway, and also loved a good challenge, I figured, "*Why not? I'll try it! A few days won't kill me.*"

I researched the different intermittent fasting patterns, and decided to try a pattern of fasting during the day, with one gigantic meal at dinner. I prepped myself mentally. I knew I was going to be simply *starving and miserable*, but hey, I could do it! I survived the initiation day on my friend's film set by chugging tea and daydreaming about the large meal I would gorge on that night. While I thought what I was doing was *crazy*, I figured it was temporary. I had committed!

The first day or so was a bit difficult, but then...

It was a breeze!

So. Easy.

I quickly fell into an effortless routine of fasting during the day and feasting at night. I also had more energy during the day, stopped stressing about meal timing, could eat all I desired at night, and slept better. Gone were the moments of thinking constantly about my next meal. It was fantastic. I was hooked. Three days soon became three years.

STAGE THREE: PALEO (c. Summer 2012)

I felt fabulous as a low carb, intermittent faster, which rendered me thin and happy. That being said, I still had my food vices. Although I had eradicated sugar, I kept my sweet tooth buzzing with artificial sweeteners, and ate processed low carb foods with their slew of toxins. When I first stumbled upon the Paleo concept one summer afternoon in my new apartment after graduating from USC, I reacted nonchalantly, thinking *"I'm doing so good already! I don't eat sugar or flour! I don't eat all day! How much of a difference can cutting out the artificial sweeteners and processed foods really make?"* However, being the health crazed self-experimenter that I am, I read Robb Wolf's *The Paleo*

Solution and decided to give Paleo a try.

The results were shocking.

Minor lingering health issues dissipated: the pain in my lower back, my Raynaud's syndrome, and my still occasional energy swings. My skin began to glow. Although low carb fasting had left me with little fat to lose at this point, the random few bits of "stubborn fat" I'd classified as part of my constitution, actually disappeared without me even trying. A few months after going Paleo, I went to the eye doctor and was shocked to find my eyesight had *improved*. I didn't know that could even be a thing.

I dived into the Paleo community with newfound enthusiasm, discovering the extensive problems stemming from what we ingest today. *(Oh hey gluten!)* I began soaking up Robb Wolf's site (robbwolf.com) and podcast ("The Paleo Solution Podcast.") I began self-experimenting with different Paleo food combinations, "superfoods," and supplements to boost performance and vitality. In a way, Paleo was my ultimate initiation into the scientific health world.

STAGE 4: WINE (c. Fall 2012)

While this last dietary element isn't really a "stage" per se, there was one more piece of the proverbial puzzle to come! You see, a miserable night of accidental overindulgence at "Film School Prom" near the end of my USC years had left me effectively unable to indulge in the stiffer stuff for a good six months. While the smell of alcohol still conjures feelings of nausea in me to this day, I did begin enjoying a glass of red wine here and there after going Paleo. (I was raised in a wine appreciating family.) I initially saw such clandestine activity as a "cheat" in my diet protocol. However, after extensive research and reading books such as Roger Corder's *The Red Wine Diet*, I realized there were a myriad of benefits from red wine consumption, arguably outweighing abstinence. I'm now a red wine girl through and through! My heart is won with wine, not chocolate.

TODAY

So here we are today. I'm a low carb Paleo, intermittent faster. People often inquire what I do to keep in "such good shape," thinking I likely starve or slave away at a gym. (I do neither.) They may also label me crazy, but I don't care. I'm never hungry during the day, nor do I stress about eating. My lifestyle yields energy, time, and productivity. I eat delicious food to complete satiety at night, and *enjoy* it. I *never* thought I'd see the day my taste buds would crave meat, vegetables, and healthy fats, yet now they do! I can easily decline bread baskets and cake - such pleasures have no power over me. When I do eat, I know the food will be used for growth, repair, and energy in my body, and will not become unnecessary and unsightly fat stores. I enjoy my glasses of wine without guilt. I feel HEALTHY inside and out. Basically, I'm a happy camper. I look back on my calorie counting, slave-to-food days and shudder.

 I'd much rather have my steak and eat it too.

IN CONSIDERATION OF CALORIES

Oh calories. The bane of existence. And yet the fuel of existence. Such irony. I debated for quite awhile on *where* to place this section exactly. In the grand scheme of Paleo and fasting things, calories are merely an afterthought. Should I tag them on at the end as clarification, or perhaps sprinkle hints throughout the book in hopes of passive-aggressively making the point? However, since calorie fixation runs rampant and can quickly derail healthy intentions, I resolved to tackle the caloric issue right from the get-go, so we can move on with our lives in a satisfactory fashion. While one could clearly write a 400+ page book on the subject, à la *Good Calories, Bad Calories* by Gary Taubes, here's a quick overview on the nature of calories, and why we all need to just calm down for a second.

WHAT IS A CALORIE?

In simplest terms, a "calorie" is a unit of heat. In the context of food, a calorie refers to how much energy a food provides. Common "diet" wisdom subscribes to the basic principle of "calories in vs. calories out." That is, if you eat less calories than you burn, you will lose weight. If you eat more calories than you burn, you will gain weight. This is an oversimplification of a true but complicated idea, often taken to erroneous conclusions. Before jumping into the nitty gritty, here are three important things to remember in regards to calories:

1. Yes, calories do matter.

2. No, not every calorie is equal.

3. If you keep your diet in line by eating the right type of foods at the right time, you probably won't need to worry much about calories at all.

Now off we go!

THE LAW OF THERMODYNAMICS

The food calorie business goes back to the whole "law of thermodynamics" conservation of energy thing. "A calorie is a calorie" adheres to the law of thermodynamics which says that energy cannot be created or destroyed. Ergo, ingested calories must be burned or stored - they cannot simply "disappear." No arguments there. Yes, if you take in more calories than you ultimately burn, you will gain weight.

It's the "amount of calories that you burn" part that throws things off. Looking at the situation in a simple "calories in vs. calories out" approach assumes the body burns a *rigid* amount of calories per day based on metabolism and exercise. It also assumes *all* calories require the same amount of energy to burn, and equally influence the body's preference for calorie burning and storing.

Therein lies the problem.

This is not the Declaration of Independence, and all calories are *not* created equal. Context is everything. The macronutrients of food (carbs, fat, protein, and alcohol) are used in a myriad of ways and affect the body's metabolism differently. Some are more readily used for structure and repair rather than fat storage. Some are hard to burn, while others are easy to store. Some encourage the body to burn fat, while others encourage it to store fat. In fact, two meals of *identical* calorie content can yield different amounts of weight loss or gain, depending on *what* they're made of and *when* they're eaten. Let's take a look at some of the different factors of calories which generate problems with the whole "calories in vs. calories out" concept.

FACTORS AFFECTING CALORIES

1. THERMIC EFFECT OF FOOD

From a pure processing standpoint, different amounts of energy are required to process different macronutrients. As noted in a 1999 *Science* article, "Energy storage efficiency can never equal unity because heat transfer is not perfect." This is known as the "thermic effect of food." Approximately 2-3% of the calories in fats, 6-8% of the calories in carbohydrates, and 25-30% of the calories in proteins are "wasted" in the digestion process. (On average, the thermic effect of a meal is credited as 10%.) This means the type of calories you eat require different amounts of energy to "eat" them in the first place. If you eat more calories from protein, for example, you will burn more calories overall than from a meal dominated by one of the other macronutrients. The calories weren't "lost," the body simply required the use of more calories for digestion and assimilation.

2. TYPES OF CALORIES

The "calories in vs. calories out" mantra does not account for the fact that different types of calories are used in different ways by the body. Consider the following examples.

Carbohydrate Calories

Carbohydrates release insulin, which *tells* your body to store fat. This means you're more likely to store than burn calories from carbs, as well as any fat calories eaten with them. Compare this to a low carb, high fat meal, which minimally affects insulin, if at all. For example, a 2009 Swedish study looked at overfeeding with carbs (in the form of candy) versus overfeeding with fat and protein (in the form of peanuts) in healthy subjects. Despite the *same* calorie intakes, only the candy group gained body fat and increased waist circumference.

Even some forms of carbs encourage more fat storage than others, as liquifying and refining carbs makes them more readily available to spike insulin and encourage fat storage. A 2010 clinical trial published in *Pharmacology, Biochemisty and Behavior*, found that rats fed high fructose corn syrup (a liquid form of fructose and glucose) gained *significantly* more weight than rats fed sucrose (a solid form of fructose and glucose), even when they consumed the *same* amount of calories. High fructose corn syrup promotes fat storage by specifically encouraging the liver to store fat. See Chapter 3: *Sweet Problems* for more on the matter.

Protein Calories
Protein is used for growth and repair in the body, rather than as a preferential energy source. While the liver can convert protein into glucose via a process called gluconeogenesis, it is a costly conversion not readily called upon. This means calories from protein are quite unlikely to contribute to fat gain, even in excess.

In fact, a 2014 *Journal of the International Society of Sports Nutrition* study found that weightlifting individuals who consumed an additional 4.4 grams of protein per pound of body weight per day (averaging an additional 800 calories per day) *did not gain weight*. As the study notes, "Certainly, this dispels the notion that 'a calorie is just a calorie'…protein calories in 'excess' of requirements are not metabolized by the body in a manner similar to carbohydrate."

MCT Calories
Consider calories from medium chain triglycerides, a type of fat abundant in coconut oil, which foregoes the typical digestion process and is instead sent directly to the liver. Since MCTs are instantly used as energy, they are not readily stored as fat. In animal trials, rats consuming the *same amount of calories* from MCT versus saturated fat lost significantly more weight when consuming MCT. Similar studies find decreased weight gain in MCT versus LCT (long chain triglyceride) diets, and decreased fat deposits in MCT versus LCT diets.

Alcohol Calories
Alcohol completely dispels the "calories in vs. calories out" theory, since the body doesn't store actual alcohol. While touted as being "high in calories" at 9 calories per gram, studies consistently show that extra calories from alcohol alone do not necessitate weight gain. A 1971 metabolic ward study found that patients gained NO weight when 1800 calories in the form of alcohol was added to their standard diet. A similar 1972 study found that substituting 50% of the patients' daily calories with alcohol yielded *weight loss*. The study also found that adding 2,000 calories of chocolate to a

patient's diet steadily increased weight, while adding 2,000 calories of alcohol negligibly affected weight.

3. TIMING OF CALORIES

Eating in restricted time windows (à la intermittent fasting, which we shall soon discuss) rather than constantly throughout the day also affects how calories are treated, setting the body's hormonal status to store less excess weight. One 2012 *Cell Metabolism* clinical trial, for example, found that mice who overate calories throughout the day gained weight, while mice who ate the *same amount of calories*, but in a restricted time window, did not. The study suggested that "the temporal feeding pattern reprograms the molecular mechanisms of energy metabolism and body weight regulation." See the *Intermittent Fasting* chapters in Part 2 for more on this.

4. BODY SET POINT

"Calories in vs. calories out" as the determining factor of weight gain and storage does not account for the body's adamant preference for homeostasis, and consequential adherence to a seeming "set point." Clinical studies of controlled calorie restriction often find that weight loss rates do not support calorie intake as the sole factor in body fat storage. Overconsumption of calories often does not yield the expected weight gain, while underconsumption often does not yield the expected weight loss. (Have you ever dieted excessively for 2 weeks yet lost seemingly nothing for your efforts? Or gone on a crazy food binge and expected to gain 5 lbs, but was back to your normal weight in a day or so? Been there, done that!)

Furthermore, weight gain can occur *without calorie overconsumption* (which is just disheartening), while weight loss can occur *without calorie reduction* (works for me!) As noted in "Body Weight Set-Points: Determination and Adjustment" (1997 *Journal of Nutrition)*, "Effects of this sort would not occur unless energy expenditure were also undergoing adjustment." In other words, the body can adjust its metabolism to account for fluctuating calorie intakes, and may raise or lower appetite to encourage homeostasis. This means that simply cutting out a few hundred calories here or there, will likely *not* instigate weight loss "over a few weeks" as often promised. (*Burn 200 calories more per day, and that's 1400 a week!* = Lies.) On the flip side, it also means that eating an extra hundred calories here or there probably won't hurt you either! Consistent long-term calorie intake, rather than day to day fluctuations, is what seems to ultimately affect the body's set point.

While the mechanisms behind the body's set point are unknown, they may involve the hypothalamus, since lesions on this part of the brain affect set weights in laboratory animal studies. The hormone leptin may also play a part in indexing the body's "energy status," instigating appropriate counter adjustments in response to shifting levels of "calorie" consumption.

Lastly, "Non-Exercise Activity Thermogenesis," or NEAT, likely plays a major role in set points. NEAT refers to all the physical activity we do which isn't conscious exercise, like fidgeting, standing up straight, or simply adding a pep to your step! NEAT can vary by up to *2,000 calories* burned per day in different individuals. For people with "good" NEAT regulation, the body will combat overeating and resist weight gain by increasing physical activity throughout the day, and resist weight loss from undereating by decreasing NEAT. A person may be completely unaware of shifting levels of NEAT. See the NEAT section in Chapter 22: *"Functional" Exercise* for more

I know for me personally, my set point has fluctuated over time in response to my evolving dietary habits. While eating a Standard American Diet in middle and early high school, I hovered around one consistent weight on the lower end of the standard BMI scale. Halfway through high school I began taking birth control for acne, and my set point shifted up by 10-20 lbs. (*Oh hey hormones!*) After adopting a low carb diet in college, it shifted back down to my earlier high school weight. Now, after implementing intermittent fasting and full-blown Paleo, my set point is actually a good 10-15 lbs lower than even that weight! These weight trends occurred over significant expanses of time, only becoming evident in retrospect.

Set points can be your worst enemy when trying to lose weight, or your best friend when you are content with it. Currently, I'm *quite* happy with my settled size, and do not fear weight gain by any means, regardless of splurges or *massive* calorie days here and there. I find it funny that I'm now a "fan" of the set point, a concept which I loathed before my low carb and intermittent fasting days. I guess set points are one reason I'm writing this book - so others can learn how to nurture their body to an easily sustainable, "set" weight they're thrilled with as well!

SO WHAT DOES IT ALL MEAN?

With calories, *context is everything*. While simple calorie counting may help you gauge your typical daily intake, calories are a highly ineffective barometer for instigating long-term weight loss. *What* you eat, and *when* you eat it, are substantially more effective factors for body weight and composition than a simple log of "calories" consumed and burned. This will be discussed thoroughly in future chapters, but basically favor protein and fat over carbs, and eat in concentrated time windows throughout the day, rather than constantly. Such eating patterns encourage fat burning and set a healthy hormonal profile of leanness, rendering calories laughably irrelevant. I cannot express enough how freeing it is to live *beyond* calories.

Part One

What?

Chapter One

What Is Paleo?

The Paleo diet refers to the prehistoric Paleolithic or "Caveman" era, but don't let the name scare you! Paleo is simply a holistic approach to health from a historical and genetic perspective, embracing whole foods on which our bodies thrive. It is not a diet fad, but rather a lifestyle. A standard Paleo diet embraces meat, vegetables, fruits, nuts, seeds, and healthy oils. It excludes grains, legumes, and any refined sugar, oil, or additives. Questionable Paleo foods include dairy, nightshades, and alcohol.

THE HISTORY STUFF

The Neolithic Revolution and introduction of agriculture around 10,000 years ago shifted society from hunting and gathering healthy whole foods we'd been consuming for thousands of years (meat, nuts, vegetables, and fruit) to inflammatory foods foreign to our bodies. Despite a complete shift in diet from the Paleolithic period, our bodies feature minimal genetic adaptations for the consumption of these new food sources. While our diet has changed massively in the last 10,000 years, our genes have not. As Boyd Eaton, an early pioneer of the Paleo approach to health, pointed out in a 1985 *New England Journal of Medicine* paper, "The human genetic constitution has changed relatively little since the appearance of truly modern human beings, Homosapiens sapiens, about 40,000 years ago. Even the development of agriculture 10,000 years ago has apparently had a minimal influence on our genes." Of course, this dietary change might not be problematic if it were an awesome, healthy and nutritious one - if refined sugar and grains were *superfoods*.

But that's just not the case.

Unfortunately, the modern diet includes nutrient-lacking, toxic grains and sugar-laden, processed concoctions which do much more harm than good. (Just wait till you get to the individual sections on these!) It's no wonder this foundational diet change heralded many of the modern diseases we have today: degenerative diseases and autoimmune conditions, diabetes and obesity, heart disease, arthritis, and even cancer. To name a few.

How can what we eat encourage disease? It may seem silly, but stick with me. Many non-Paleo "foods" wreck havoc on the digestive system, inhibiting nutrient absorption and instigating systemic inflammation. This plunges the body into a state of panic, resulting in autoimmune diseases in which the body confuses "invader" proteins with its *own* proteins, and creates antibodies against itself. (Talk about shooting yourself in the foot!) Non-Paleo foods also cause insulin levels to skyrocket, which promotes fat storage, diabetes, obesity, and all the problems arriving with such.

Let's break things down a bit, shall we? (No pun intended.)

WHAT IS DISEASE?

"Disease" refers to maladies suffered by the body. Two major types of diseases are *infectious diseases* from external sources, and *degenerative diseases* which originate within the body.

Infectious diseases come from pesky pathogens like viruses, bacteria, and fungi. Examples of infectious diseases include the common cold, flu, measles, and chicken pox. (If you want to get dark and historical, think the bubonic plague or Ebola virus.) Infectious diseases are prevented and treated by vaccines, as well as a healthy, properly functioning immune system.

Degenerative diseases are more complex, involving the deterioration of body tissues and organs. They basically come from "broken machinery" within the body — when cells stop functioning correctly. Degenerative diseases are discouraged via preventative lifestyle measures to ensure the "equipment" doesn't break in the first place. Ironically, degenerative diseases can actually be exacerbated by an overactive immune system. (More on that later.) Common degenerative diseases include arthritis, diabetes, Alzheimer's, and heart disease. A prime example of degenerative disease is cancer, in which malignant cells with genetic defects reproduce at an expedited rate, overwhelming the body and interfering with key essential functions. Only a small percentage of cancer cases are inherited, while 90-95% of cancer occurrences are linked to lifestyle choices. 30-35% of deaths from cancer are linked to diet.

But I'm getting ahead of myself.

THE CONNECTION BETWEEN FOOD AND DISEASE
Observational studies indicate degenerative diseases likely stem from lifestyle choices rather than genetics. For example, chronic illness is influenced more by the country one lives in, rather than the country one is from. Similarly, twin studies insinuate genes typically do not determine illness. A person is not necessarily "born with" a future of arthritis, diabetes, or stroke. The choices we make in how we live (including diet, exercise, and environment) may be the defining factor in our overall heath.

In today's society, we like to apply the first type of disease model discussed, infectious disease, to all bodily dysfunction. We readily attribute health problems to some third party invader, fixed by popping a third party pill. This view of the body sees the symptoms as the problem to be fixed, rather than addressing the greater underlying condition. In contrast, a holistic view of the body and disease, like the Paleo perspective, interprets the majority of ailments as *signs* of a deeper overarching problem within the body. The foundational "source problem," whatever it may be, is often inflammatory and autoimmune in nature - a state created by the body reacting to foreign, toxic substances in our diet.

WHAT IS INFLAMMATION?
Inflammation gets a bad rap all around, although it bears good intentions in spirit. Inflammation is actually a protective process

which allows an infected area to heal. The word comes from the Latin "inflammare," meaning "to set on fire"…which is kind of what it does. Inflammation is the body's reaction to trouble. When reactive proteins in the body called "pattern recognition receptors" (PRRs) sense an injury or pathogen, they initiate the "inflamed" state you likely know well: redness, swelling, increased temperature, reduced function, and pain. Fun times. A common sign of inflammation is high levels of a PRR called C-reactive protein (CRP).

Although unpleasant to experience, the inflamed state is a healthy, healing process… in theory. The problems begin when we shift from injury-based *acute inflammation* (like a stubbed toe), to prolonged *chronic inflammation*. This second type of inflammation occurs when the body enters an inflamed state and begins needlessly instigating prolonged inflammatory responses. Rather than attacking the invader or healing an injury, the body attacks itself. Chronic inflammation can range from the unpleasant but relatively benign (like skin rashes or inflammatory bowel disease), to the more serious and even life-threatening (like rheumatoid arthritis, Celiac disease, or heart disease). Even cancer is linked to inflammation.

THE MODERN RESPONSE TO INFLAMMATION: PAIN PILLS

As far back as elementary school, I was intrigued by aspirin. I found it suspicious that one pill could miraculously fix any painful ailment. It simply didn't make sense to me. Shouldn't there be *separate* headache pills, stubbed toe pills, sprain pills, and sore pills? How could one pill address *everything*? Although I'd ask grown-ups this question, I never received a satisfactory answer. Until now.

Over-the-counter pain pills such as aspirin, Advil, and Aleve are categorized as NSAIDs: non-steroidal anti-inflammatory drugs. NSAIDs work by blocking enzymes (like Cox-1 and Cox-2) in charge of releasing the hormones which green-light the inflammation. NSAIDs can "stop" the inflammation response from ever occurring in the first place. While seemingly great as a temporary fix, NSAIDs only mask the problem. They do not solve nor, dare I say, even address it.

Popping a pill to calm down inflammation doesn't fix the actual issue - the "why" of the situation. Wouldn't it be better to stop the cause of inflammation in the first place, rather than silence the body's response to it? Beyond that, NSAIDs increase intestinal permeability within 24 hours of ingestion, which actually *encourages* inflammation.

In short term studies, NSAIDs create erythema (redness from inflammation) and potential ulcers. Long-term studies of their use find *bleeding* stomach ulcers and NSAID-induced enteropathy (inflammation of the intestines). Such irony.

FOOD AND INFLAMMATION

Modern food choices like sugar, grains, and processed foods, majorly encourage the body's overreactive, inflammatory state. They wreck havoc on our bodies, which register them as toxins and initiate the immune response. This can escalate to the point that the body begins attacking itself in the process of trying to kill the toxic "invader." Sad day.

Let's take a look at the big inflammatory *no no's* of Paleo, all which became food sources in relatively recent human industry: *grains* (which contain problematic proteins and toxic anti-nutrients), *refined sugar* (which is highly inflammatory and spikes insulin, encouraging fat storage), and *processed foods* (which contain straight-up toxins).

Chapter Two

Grainy Problems

Grains are the seeds of grasses, and include three of the world's top crops: rice, wheat, and maize. Other grains include oats, barley, cornmeal, millet, and sorghum. A grain is composed of the *germ*, *endosperm*, and *bran*. The germ is the living embryo of the grain, featuring most of its nutrients. The endosperm provides energy for the germ, and is made of starch and protein. The bran is the hard, protective outer layer of the grain, containing fiber and B vitamins.

Whole grains, like whole wheat flour and brown rice, contain the germ, endosperm, and bran. *Refined grains*, like white flour and white rice, have been processed to remove the bran and germ, leaving only the starchy endosperm. Many refined grains are artificially "enriched" with vitamins, since the refining process strips them of most nutrients. Whole grains are touted as "healthy" because they contain the original vitamins, minerals, and fiber found in the germ and bran. However, they also contain more of the plant's anti-nutrients, which we shall discuss. (Get excited!)

Grains are the foundation of the world's food source today. Highly economical, grains have supported the industrial and technological achievements of mankind, since you arguably must eat to do productive things. So that's good.

Except that's where the good ends.

THE TOXIC NATURE OF GRAINS

When attacked or facing danger, living things tend to either assume the offensive and fight back, or favor the defensive by raising shields or running away. (I prefer the defensive *build-a-tent-and-camp-out* method myself.) But *plants* are in a proverbial pickle, since they can't attack or run away. So what do they do? Simple.

Become super passive aggressive.

In order to discourage being consumed, plants contain *anti-nutrient compounds* which serve as a silent but deadly defense mechanism: you eat the plant and experience ill digestive side effects (and hopefully learn from your mistakes). Sure, the plant still dies for the cause, but its ghost haunts your memory. These protective mechanisms also potentially protect the seed from digestion, so perhaps the seed can *still* survive after wrecking havoc on your digestive tract. Double win. (This is a bit different from fruit-bearing plants, which allure us with their sweetness and *count* on being eaten to spread their seed.)

The anti-nutrient compounds particularly abundant in grains include *gluten, lectins,* and *phytates.* Other problematic plant compounds include *saponins, goitrogens, oxalates,* and *protease inhibitors,* to name a few. If you're wondering, the whole "soaking" and "sprouting" trend is an effort to deactivate the toxic parts of the grain. Now you can walk by the sprouted section at Whole Foods with a smug "knowingness."

GLUTEN

When I found out I was allergic to wheat, I jumped for joy. It was like my official invitation to the gluten-free club. GF for the win! I was no longer the "poser" I felt like up until that point. (*"Hi! I don't eat gluten because...umm...it's bad. Can I sit with you guys?"*)

Chances are, you've heard a bit about this nefarious "gluten." It seems the low fat craze is slowly succumbing to the gluten-free craze. (Thank goodness.) But what exactly is this nebulous grain anti-nutrient called gluten? And what's the difference between gluten sensitivity, allergies, and Celiac? Just what is happening? Is this a craze or a real thing? Let's take a walk down Gluten Avenue!

Gluten is a large protein storage molecule found in grains. It is the main structural protein in wheat, the world's most widely grown crop. It also makes an appearance in other cereal grains such as rye and barley. Many of today's wheat products have been technologically engineered to contain more protein, and thus more gluten along with it. Lovely.

Gluten also makes its way into most processed foods. Gluten gives bread extra chewiness, is used as a stabilizing agent, and serves as an additive for protein. Basically, gluten is everywhere. Sneaky devil. *"I didn't know BBQ sauce would have gluten,"* said my sister, when I offered her some gluten-free BBQ sauce. Yep. If it comes in a package and doesn't say "gluten-free," just assume a bit of gluten lurks inside.

Gluten is difficult for the body to digest, and contains a toxic compound called *gliadin*. Gliadin is completely resistant to digestion by enzymes within the body. In vitro studies show gliadin wreaks havoc on cells, even *before* any allergic or immune response: it binds to things, inhibits cell growth, increases intestinal permeability, rearranges the cytoskeleton, alters enzymes in the esophagus, and even instigates apoptosis (programmed cell death, AKA cell suicide).

Gluten commonly yields digestive issues such as gas, bloating, and irritable bowel syndrome (IBS). It can also create intestinal permeability, allowing food particles and toxins to leak into the bloodstream, a condition known as "Leaky Gut Syndrome." Gluten easily sparks an immune response, causing the body to attack the gluten particles, and itself in the process. Associated issues from this impaired digestion and/or leaky gut include digestive issues, skin problems, fatigue, and irritability on the more benign end, to more serious conditions like rheumatoid arthritis, osteoporosis, and even cancer. Gluten has also been linked to psychiatric and neurological diseases such as depression, dementia, autism, epilepsy, and schizophrenia.

The nomenclature regarding gluten-related problems is widely debated. I shall break it down into 4 categories: *Wheat Allergy, Celiac Disease, Gluten Sensitivity,* and the *"Non-Sensitive."* While sharing similar symptoms, the mechanism of action, timing, and severity may differ.

1. Wheat Allergy
For those allergic to wheat (likely due to the gluten), the body

initiates an immune response releasing IgE antibodies when it comes in contact with wheat. Symptoms may occur rather immediately, within minutes to hours. Wheat allergies vary in nature, although they may occur through food (dietary allergy), inhalation (baker's asthma), contact (contact urticaria), or even from exercise after wheat consumption (wheat-dependent exercise-induced anaphylaxis). I find that last one fascinating.

For those allergic to gluten, the immune response may lead to a variety of issues: skin (hives, rashes, eczema, dermatitis), gastrointestinal (digestive problems, gas, bloating), or respiratory (throat problems, voice issues, asthma). In extreme cases, a wheat allergy may result in fatal anaphylaxis.

Population surveys are conflicting, but wheat allergies seem to occur more commonly in children (4-9%), and decrease with age (around .5-3% of adults). Like I said, I have a wheat allergy, and the blood test to prove it!

2. Celiac Disease

Beyond wheat allergy lies the darker, crème de la crème gluten reaction: Celiac disease. With this autoimmune disease, the body mounts an intense immune response to gluten, ultimately resulting in enteropathy (inflammation of the intestines). It typically takes weeks to years after gluten exposure for the effects to become apparent, although some Celiac patients do react immediately with diarrhea, nausea, or other digestive problems.

An inflamed intestine inhibits nutrient absorption and can result in intestinal problems like diarrhea, gas, bloating, vomiting, constipation, and malabsorption, as well as extra-intestinal symptoms such as malnutrition, fatigue, skin problems, anemia, osteoporosis, neurological disturbances, memory problems, infertility, cancer, and even death.

Approximately 1% of the population suffers from Celiac disease, although recent studies indicate the percentage is rising, likely due to the global increase of wheat consumption. Sad day. (Although the fact that this trend encourages research on Celiac disease is a silver lining.)

3. Gluten Sensitivity

Approximately 10% of the population is estimated to be "gluten sensitive," meaning they suffer an immune reaction to gluten, without an apparent allergic or autoimmune component. Those who are gluten sensitive may experience symptoms similar to those with a wheat allergy or Celiac disease, hours to days after exposure: digestive issues, abdominal pain, diarrhea, headache, bone or joint pain, muscle cramps, numbness, fatigue, "foggy mind," depression, anemia, etc.

4. The "Non-Sensitive"

Ok, this one is kind of a trick. Even if you're not *specifically* sensitive or allergic to gluten by "technical" standards, gluten maintains its sinister nature. Gluten contains at least 50 epitopes (like the aforementioned gliadin) which instigate T-cell responses (an immune reaction). As a 2011 *BMC Medicine* review of gluten notes, "All individuals, even those with a low degree of risk, are... susceptible to some form of gluten reaction during their life span."

So What Does It All Mean?

Clearly, gluten is bad stuff. However, you don't have to live in fear! Whatever gluten clique you call home (Wheat Allergy, Celiac, Gluten-Sensitive, or Non-Sensitive), a gluten-free diet prevents all the problems of gluten! (Surprise, surprise.) And of course, a Paleo diet is by nature gluten-free. Avoid the grains and bread at all cost, as well as processed foods. Look for "gluten-free" labels. Luckily, gluten-free is increasingly gaining popularity: in 2010, the gluten-free global market reached almost $2.5 billion (US) in sales. And since the current zeitgeist labels gluten-free *in vogue,* you can confidently parade around the store with your gluten-free content laden cart, to the envy of onlookers!

LECTINS

As the Scarecrow says en route to Oz, *"I think it'll get darker before it gets lighter."* That's right folks: if the whole gluten thing was making you a little nervous, it gets worse! Gluten has an even more nefarious cousin lurking in the corner, named *Lectin.* Everyone introduce yourself!

Lectins are a protein found in plants, functioning as a part of the plant's natural defense mechanism. They're particularly concentrated in grains - primarily wheat, but also rye and barley. Furthermore, lectins are found in legumes and tubers such as potatoes, beans, and soy. Lectins are notably resilient to cooking and digestive enzymes. No avoiding these little buggers.

Oh, and a lectin's sole purpose is to destroy you. Kind of.

The word "lectin" comes from the Latin word "legere," meaning "to select." Lectins are particularly "sticky" proteins which bind to sugar molecules to ward off invaders. If a bacteria, virus, or fungus comes around, the toxic lectins "select" and attach to the invader's sugary membrane in order to deter and destroy it. Lectins are extremely efficient in warding off fungi. That makes them pretty strong stuff in my opinion.

If *you* ingest lectins, they don't lose their sticky fancy for sugar. This is bad news for your digestive tract, since the intestinal wall is composed of epithelial cells containing, you guessed it, sugars! Lectins attach to the intestinal wall and can cause intestinal damage, leading to an array of nasty problems, like indigestion, nausea, and diarrhea. They strip away the protective mucous layer in the stomach and intestines, stimulate acid secretion, bind to immune cells, and inhibit repair of damaged cells in general, be it from themselves or any other cause. Lectins can do all of this damage directly to cells and tissue: no prior allergy, intolerance, or autoimmune condition required!

Lectins are also considered anti-nutrients because, in binding to everything, they prevent absorption of *actual* nutrients. So not only do lectins wreak havoc of their own accord, they also simultaneously prevent the body from receiving the nutrients needed to fight back, or deal with any other health issues. Lectins attack offensively, while shattering the body's defense. Double whammy. If this were football, you'd probably want to be on team Lectin.

And if all this weren't bad enough, lectins can permeate the intestinal wall and enter the bloodstream, binding to anything and everything, while leeching minerals and creating systemic inflammation. These holes created in the digestive track can allow bacteria and bits of food to enter the bloodstream, yielding the aforementioned "leaky gut syndrome." When the body senses these leaked foreign invaders in the bloodstream, it creates antibodies and mounts an immune response. In doing so, the body often injures itself in the process of attacking the lectin-clad cells. This can lead to a slew of issues like allergies, fatigue, skin rashes, and joint inflammation. And while the body is stressed by dealing with all this madness, other simple body tasks like digestion can fall by the wayside. Oh hey IBS, constipation, and diarrhea!

With their resilient maliciousness, it's no surprise that lectins are

linked to metabolic syndrome, obesity, arthritis, and many other chronic diseases. Lectins can also bind to thyroid nodules, as well as cross the blood-brain barrier and cause inflammation in the brain, leading to neurological diseases.
To round out the lectin picture, let's zero in on one particularly nasty and abundant lectin: *wheat germ agglutinin*. Wheat germ agglutinin (WGA) is found in wheat (shocker), and actually gives gluten some lectin activity. WGA is so efficient at destroying invaders, that wheat is currently being engineered to *increase* WGA content in order to function as a "natural" pesticide. Of course, this means there's more WGA to go around in your system once you eat this wheat. Awesome. (Not really.) In clinical trials, WGA has been shown to bind to the cells of the small intestine, interfere with the gut, alter metabolism, permeate the gut wall into circulation, integrate into blood vessel walls, bind to immune cells, instigate pro-inflammatory cytokines, cause atrophy of the thymus, inhibit nuclear DNA replication, bind to nerve fibers, and affect the central nervous system. And like lectins in general, WGA can do direct harm to cells even if the person is neither allergic nor sensitive to wheat.

PHYTATES

Phytates are found primarily in grains, legumes, nuts, and seeds (with highest concentrations in whole grains and beans). On the plus side, phytates can function as antioxidants with potential anti-cancer properties. However, phytic acid (the main component of a phytate) is an anti-nutrient, and can bind to minerals in the body such as calcium, magnesium, zinc, iron, and phosphorous, preventing their absorption. While phytates are likely only problematic if you're consuming large amounts of beans and/or whole grains {cough} *Grain-Based FDA Pyramid* {cough}, I vote erring on the side of less rather than more.

OTHER GRAINY PROBLEMS

Besides gluten, lectins, and phytates, grains feature a few other nasty characteristics.

1. High GI

Grains are high on the *glycemic index*: a measure of the extent to which a certain food raises blood sugar. As such, grains quickly elevate blood sugar and release insulin, which spikes appetite and fat storage. (See the next chapter, *Sweet Problems* for more on that.) Both white bread and wheat bread have similar GIs, averaging in the low 70s. For comparison, a Coca Cola averages to 63, and a Snickers Bar is a 51. In an extensive test of the glycemic index of whole foods, cereal grains (particularly breakfast cereals), legumes like beans and peas, and potatoes elevated blood sugar levels the most.

2. FODMAPs

Grains are high in FODMAPs: compounds which are highly fermentable, but difficult to absorb by the small intestine. They can sit around in your gut and ferment, encouraging gastrointestinal distress. Some people are particularly sensitive to FODMAPs, and may need to specifically restrict them. Furthermore, many people suffer from an overgrowth of bacteria in the small intestine, a condition called SIBO. SIBO is common because the modern overuse of antibiotics easily wipes out the "good bacteria" in the digestive tract, allowing bad bacteria to flourish. If you have SIBO, FODMAPs may serve as food for these nasty little buggers, and the toxins they produce after consuming FODMAPS can make you feel pretty terrible. For more on the gut microbiome, consider reading David Perlmutter's *Brain Maker: The Power of Gut Microbes To Heal And Protect Your Brain - For Life*.

3. Opioid-Like Peptides

Grains contain peptides which may give them opioid-like, addictive qualities, and even instigate behavioral changes. One theory even links the opioid activity in grains to schizophrenia, which is around 30 times more prevalent in people with Celiac. So your intense hankering for bread may actually just be a sign of opiate withdrawal - no big deal.

4. Alpha-Amylase Inhibitors

Alpha-amylase inhibitors serve as a defense mechanism in grains primarily against insects. They are an allergen for some people, specifically in "baker's asthma." They also inhibit digestive enzymes produced by the pancreas for starch. On the one hand, this can reduce insulin spikes, and the compound is actually sold commercially in "carb blocking" supplements such as Phase 2. (Which I may or may not have tried back in my low carb, pre-Paleo days.) However, animal studies on long-term alpha-amylase inhibitors administration show adverse effects on the pancreas, making these compounds iffy stuff.

5. Protease Inhibitors

Like alpha-amylase inhibitors, protease inhibitors also inhibit digestive enzymes, specifically one called trypsin. In animal studies, this causes the pancreas to release too much cholecystokinin, resulting in hypertrophy of the pancreas and encouraging cancer.

6. Insufficient Protein Content

Protein content in grains averages around 12%, while protein content of meat averages around 22%. Unlike the complete protein content of meat (featuring all 9 amino acids in sufficient quantities), grains tend to be incomplete, providing insufficient amounts of lysine and threonine. This means you need to consume even *more* grains to provide adequate protein intake in a grain-based diet. And that's just no bueno.

7. Poor in Nutrients

Grains display a feeble pallor on the nutritional scale. They contain no vitamin A, vitamin C, or carotenoids, and are low in antioxidants. While grains do contain the majority of B vitamins, they lack the pivotal vitamin B12. B12 deficiencies often lead to energy problems such as weakness, tiredness, or light-headedness on the more benign end, and anemia on the more serious end. Furthermore, the bioavailability of B vitamins in grains is quite low, especially compared to their high bioavailability in meat. Nutrient deficiencies associated with increased grain consumption include biotin, niacin, the amino acid tryptophan, and thiamin.

Studies show high grain intake inhibits Vitamin D metabolism, although the actual mechanisms are unclear. And while whole grains do feature iron, zinc, and copper, their bioavailability is low, due to fiber and phytate content. Grains are low in calcium but high in phosphorous and magnesium, which yields unfavorable ratios. Low calcium is just a bad thing all around, and while phosphorous is "good," high phosphorous intake coupled with low calcium intake negatively affects metabolism and bone density. Furthermore, the unfavorable calcium/magnesium ratio in grains encourages calcium excretion. Diets with a foundation of grains correlate to higher rates of osteomalacia, rickets, and osteoporosis.

While one can argue obtaining these missing nutrients from

other food sources, grains tend to *replace* meat, fruit, and vegetables in one's diet, rather than *supplement* them. It's no wonder a myriad of studies link grain based diets to nutritional deficiencies, even though many grain products are now "fortified" with extra vitamins. And while "whole grains" may contain more nutrients than "refined grains," they also contain more problematic anti-nutrients. Ya just can't win.

WHAT ABOUT FIBER?

Let's zero in on fiber for a second. Fiber refers to indigestible carbohydrates found in the cell walls of plants. It adds no real caloric or nutritional value to food, but can serve as a bulking agent ("filling you up," so to speak), regulate digestion, and feed gut flora. (Fiber can make you gassy because the bacteria in your gut produce gas when they digest fiber.) Fiber can be either *soluble*, meaning it dissolves in water, or *insoluble*, meaning it does not. Soluble fiber tends to bulk up in your system, while insoluble fiber basically passes through unchanged.

While not as deleterious to health as the low fat paradigm discussed in Chapter 5: *Fat Problems*, the whole "eat more fiber thing" is a bit misleading. I like to think of fiber as a reality TV star: quite famous, but of questionable merit. Our dear friend fiber first joined the popular crowd in the 1960s, when British surgeon Dennis Burkitt theorized that it protected against colon cancer. While studying lymphoma cancer affecting children in East Africa, Burkitt noticed that certain cancers prevalent in Western civilization were notably absent in poor, third world countries. He compared the indigenous populations' *whole food* diets featuring fibrous fruit and vegetables, to the Western diet of refined flour and sugar, and concluded it was the *lack of fiber* in the refined diet which prevented colon cancer, rather than any other difference between the diets. (Perhaps the *addition* of refined sugar and carbohydrates?) Burkitt wrote a book on his findings (with no concrete supportive studies), and fiber became a legend. As Gary Taubes says in *Good Calories, Bad Calories,* "Better to say 'Don't Forget Fibre in Your Diet,' which was the title of Burkitt's 1979 diet book, than to say 'Don't eat sugar, flour, and white rice, and drink less beer.'"

Ok, so fiber's rise to fame was based on an assumption, but surely studies later confirmed its health benefits, right?

Not so much.

A 2007 review of fiber studies entitled "Primary dietary prevention: is the fiber story over?" noted the conflicting nature of such studies, concluding that the relation between fiber and colon cancer has not been adequately addressed, with further trials and research needed. That's a lot of grey area for an "eat more fiber" mantra saturating a nation and fueling the sale of commercial products. More recently, a 2000 *New England Journal of Medicine* study evaluating the use of cereal bran fiber in 1429 patients concluded that "a dietary supplement of wheat-bran fiber does not protect against recurrent colorectal adenomas," which are the precursors for colon cancer. Shortly thereafter, a follow-up study in 2002 re-evaluated 1208 of the original patients, just in case they weren't *actually* eating enough fiber... and reached the same conclusion:

> The results of this study show that neither fiber intake from a wheat bran supplement nor total fiber intake affects the recurrence of colorectal adenomas, thus lending further evidence to the body of literature indicating that consumption of a high-fiber diet, especially one rich in cereal fiber, does not reduce the risk of colorectal adenoma recurrence.

Not only is fiber's merits questionable, but excess fiber may even be detrimental. Back in 1979, a study found that, while a high animal protein (i.e.: meat) diet had no effect on colon cancer as suspected, adding fiber actually *increased* calcium excretion despite an increase in calcium intake. Besides calcium, excess fiber may also bind to other minerals such as magnesium and iron, making them less absorbable.

As noted in the 2003 *Journal of Pediatric Gastroenterology & Nutrition*, potential risks of too much fiber in young children include maldigestion, malabsoprtion, and stunted growth. And while the commentary notes that fiber may encourage insulin sensitivity and discourage childhood obesity, the reasoning is that added fiber reduces "excessive intakes of energy-dense, sweet, and fat-rich foods and drinks." Like Burkitt's theory, fiber is once again heralded as "protective" when, in reality, it may be the *other* added foods like sugar and refined carbs which are actually causing the problem. A 2007 *World Journal of Gastroenterology* review nicely summarizes fiber's controversial history, and concludes:

> Whilst it is not the intention of the authors to totally discourage fiber in the diet and the use of fiber supplements, there does not seem to be much use for fiber in colorectal diseases. We, however, want to emphasize that what we have all been made to believe about fiber needs a second look. We often choose to believe a lie, as a lie repeated often enough by enough people becomes accepted as the truth. We urge clinicians to keep an open mind. While there are some benefits of a diet high in natural fiber, one must know the exact indications before recommending such a diet. Myths about fiber must be debunked and truth installed.

I as well am not saying fiber is a "bad" thing, merely that its benefits may be overhyped. But if you're still worried about getting enough fiber on a Paleo diet, or perhaps find a certain amount of pristine pride in your fiber-induced bathroom yule logs, there's no need to fret! Calorie for calorie, the amount of fiber in green vegetables far outweighs that of grains, and can provide all of fiber's benefits without the grainy health assault. On a 100 calorie basis, bread contains around 1.5-3 grams of fiber, while green vegetables such as broccoli, spinach, and lettuce, contain 7-10 grams. Paleo foods high in fiber include green vegetables, squash, sweet potatoes, avocados, and fruits such as apples and berries. As for the fruits, stripping them of their fiber à la juicing or dehydration only serves to increase their glycemic index and raise insulin levels. Don't do it.

SO WHAT DOES IT ALL MEAN?

Grains are disagreeable for two main reasons:

1. Grains wreak havoc on your gut, leading to a myriad of diseases.

2. By forming the foundation of a diet, grains replace nutritious food and encourage deficiencies.

With everything bad going for them, grains just don't have much good going for them. They're cheap and economical. That's pretty much it. Given the toxic nature of grains, coupled with their lack of benefits, it's no surprise that a grain-based diet poses quite a few problems. I'm looking at you FDA food pyramid!

Chapter Three

Sweet Problems

"Sugar" is a general term referring to the sweet stuff we get from simple and complex carbohydrates. *Simple carbohydrates* are "simple" molecules of sugar, like you find in table sugar or refined flour. They break down very quickly in the body, spiking blood sugar. *Complex carbohydrates* are chains of sugar molecules found in starches like sweet potatoes, tubers, and whole grains. They take longer for the body to break down and affect blood sugar at a more "steady" rate.

The rate at which a certain carbohydrate affects blood sugar is measured by the glycemic index (GI), a scale of 0-100. Pure glucose dissolved in water is 100. Since simple carbohydrates are quickly digested, they have higher GIs. Complex carbohydrates dissolve more slowly, and fall lower on the scale. Anything that speeds up digestion of the sugar in a food will raise its GI, like refining flour, dehydrating fruit, or juicing vegetables. Fat and protein in a food tend to lower the GI, although studies show that a mixed meal of fat, protein, and carbohydrates can still yield a high GI if the net intake of carbs is high enough.

Here are two essential points about this whole carbohydrate/sugar thing which just might blow your mind:

1. Every carbohydrate you ingest *regardless of the original source* (candy, cereal, bread, pasta, potatoes, rice, fruit, vegetables, etc.) is ultimately converted into *blood sugar* (glucose). Even if you eat a piece of broccoli, that broccoli will partly become blood sugar, albeit a relatively negligible bit.

2. Although commonly used and intensely monitored by the body, there is no actual *requirement* for carbohydrates. Our body can generate the minimal amount of glucose it needs from protein and fat (if necessary) via a process called gluconeogenesis. However, it *cannot* generate protein or fat (the foundation of the body) from any other substrate.

SUGAR AND YOUR BODY

Let's look at simple carbohydrates (AKA plain ol' sugar). The three main types of simple sugar are *glucose*, *fructose*, and *sucrose*. All of these are ultimately converted into glucose ("blood sugar") by the body. (With the exception of some tricky business involving fructose, to be discussed later.)

Glucose is a fuel, which is a good thing. On the flip side, too much glucose is actually toxic to the body. An unprocessed whole foods diet effectively moderates blood sugar, minimizing damage. Our modern diet rampant in added and refined sugar, however, is a different story.

Here are just a few of sugar's sticky problems:

1. Red Blood Cells and Cholesterol

Think about the sugar you're likely most familiar with: white table sugar. It's sticky stuff, right? It's therefore not surprising that high concentrations of sugar in the blood can stick to red blood cells, interfering with circulation and causing the fat molecule "cholesterol" to rise. Yep, it's not the fat which causes high cholesterol and all the associated problems - it's the sugar!

2. Glycation and Free-Radicals

Sugar can also stick to proteins in a process called *glycation*. Glycation instigates inflammation and increases *free-radicals* by 50 fold.

Here's a vast oversimplification of the free-radical concept. The cells in your body constantly react with oxygen, which can lead to the nasty little free-radicals. A free-radical is like a *super needy, clingy friend* who also happens to just be a mean person in general. Free-radicals run around the body looking for other cells to "react" with, and then damage their membranes, proteins, and genes. As such, glycation is directly correlated to aging and deterioration of the body. If I were to say that "too many carbs = death," that would seem like crazy talk. Except they kinda do… or at least point the body in that direction.

3. Inflammation

Sugar is highly inflammatory and increases blood levels of inflammatory cytokines. Check out Chapter 1: *What Is Paleo?* for more about inflammation.

4. Hampered Immune System

Sugar disables phagocytosis in white blood cells, which is their protective capacity to engulf foreign particles, bacteria, and invaders. It's how they "eat" and expunge toxic things. Consuming more sugar therefore encourages an accumulation of toxins in the body.

5. Oxidative Stress

Sugar raises levels of oxidative stress, which refers to the whole free-radical business mentioned in #2. (The rebellious little molecules in the body searching for electrons, which attach to *healthy* cells and wreck havoc.) Increased oxidative stress is linked to tissue damage and diseases like cancer and Alzheimers. Antioxidants are protective against oxidative stress. *(Can I get some red wine over here?)* Sugar, on the other hand, just aggravates the matter.

6. Addiction

Similar to drugs, sugar instigates addictive behavior by releasing dopamine and opioids. In clinical trials, rats can become sugar-dependent. So when you're casually like, *"I'm addicted to sugar!,"* well… maybe it's not so casual.

7. Cancer

Cancer cells feed on sugar, and sugar intake is strongly correlated with many forms of cancer. In fact, doctors are now using glucose injections to *find* cancerous cells in the body. Furthermore, sugarless ketogenic diets (discussed in the *Intermittent Fasting* chapters), are actively being studied as a dietary method for putting cancer into remission.

8. Insulin

Perhaps sugar's biggest issue, especially in our present day carbohydrate-fueled society, is its relationship to insulin, fueling diabetes and obesity through insulin resistance.

SUGAR AND INSULIN

To understand how a high carbohydrate (i.e.: sugar) diet hinders weight loss and adversely affects health in general, we must first understand the relationship between sugar and insulin levels.

Insulin is a hormone in the body responsible for transporting nutrients from your food into cells. It is also the primary regulator of fat storage. When you eat carbs, their sugar elevates your blood sugar levels. (This is unlike protein and fat, which minimally affect blood sugar.) Since too much sugar in the body is toxic, as previously discussed, the pancreas produces insulin to move the sugar into cells throughout the body. As such, insulin "shuts off" fat burning and promotes fat storage. Insulin is a good thing because it lowers blood sugar and assimilates nutrients, but things get tricky. (Don't they always?)

Insulin works "correctly" when we eat whole foods which moderately affect blood sugar levels, keeping all hormones and body functions in check: blood sugar rises after we eat some carbs, insulin takes care of it, and everyone's a happy camper! Modern processed foods high in refined sugar, however, *rapidly* raise blood sugar and encourage insulin release far beyond levels to which the body is accustomed. From there, things just get gnarly.

Here's how it goes down.

Carbohydrates (AKA: sugar) get turned into glucose in the bloodstream, causing blood sugar to rise. The pancreas senses this rise and releases insulin to shuttle the glucose to its temporary storage place: as glycogen in muscles and the liver. Now, in the good ol' days of limited carbohydrates, this was all fine and dandy. Today, however, with our high sugar intake and often sedentary lifestyles, the glycogen stores in the muscles and liver are often full. So insulin takes glucose to the backup plan: fat stores! Yep. Sugar becomes fat. And it can get worse…

INSULIN RESISTANCE

Constant sugar and insulin barraging the cells throughout the body can make them *less* sensitive to insulin. *Insulin resistance* occurs when normal amounts of insulin become insufficient to shuttle glucose into cells. The cells basically get tired of being hit with insulin all the time, so they downregulate their insulin receptors. It's like when kids put their hands over their ears and say, *"I'm not listening!"* Since the glucose can't get into these "stubborn" cells, blood sugar remains elevated. So the pancreas is like *"OMG! Toxic blood sugar is still high!"* and produces *more* insulin to lower blood sugar. Since insulin is the regulator and instigator of fat storage, increasingly high levels of insulin from insulin resistance puts the body into a constant fat-storing mode.

What's ironic about this whole situation, is that the body is actively storing nutrients in fat cells, but may still "believe" it is starving. Since the stubborn cells, resistant to accepting glucose from insulin, are not receiving their fuel, the brain instigates a ravenous appetite to eat more, even when too much has already been consumed. Hello never-ending spiral into simultaneous hunger and fat gain!

Insulin resistance can lead to the metabolic syndrome and obesity, while the wear and tear on the pancreas from constant insulin production can instigate Type II diabetes. (Type I diabetes is typically genetic and occurs when the person lacks the ability to produce insulin, while Type II diabetes signifies insufficient use of insulin and is developed from lifestyle.) In fact, an extensive 2013 epidemiological study found that the availability of sugar statistically determines diabetes rates. As stated in *PLoS ONE*:

> Sugar availability appears to be uniquely correlated to diabetes prevalence independent of overweight and obesity prevalence rates, unlike other food types and total consumption, and independent of other changes in economic and social change such as urbanization, aging, changes to household income, sedentary lifestyles, and tobacco or alcohol use.

In other words, sugar consumption alone, regardless of other factors, correlates strongest to diabetes.

PALEO AND INSULIN SENSITIVITY

But not to fear! Paleo moderates blood sugar levels because it is devoid of insulin-spiking, sugar-laden foods. A Paleo diet is rich in protein and fat, which do not significantly raise blood sugar levels, while fruit and vegetables contain substantially less sugar than processed foods, and are typically rich in water and fiber which slows sugar release.

By moderating blood sugar levels on a lower carb diet (especially compared to modern standards), Paleo encourages *insulin sensitivity*: a state in which insulin does its job properly, efficiently utilizing sugar and nutrients from food, without endless appetite, fat gain, and the problems arising from such. Without excess insulin promoting fat storage, the body also relies more on fat stores for fuel, which is awesome for both body composition and health in general.

TYPES OF SUGAR

The most basic sugars are the simple sugars *glucose* and *fructose*, as well as their combined disaccharide form of *sucrose*. Other sugars include *maltose* (a disaccharide of two glucose) and *lactose* (a disaccharide of glucose and galactose).

1. Glucose

Glucose is a *monosaccharide*, or single unit sugar. As discussed, most carbohydrates you eat are processed into glucose in the body, where it becomes "blood sugar." Glucose is found primarily in vegetables, nuts, and grains. It's often "starchy." It can be used immediately for energy, or stored as glycogen in the muscles and liver. When glycogen stores are filled, excess glucose is stored as fat in cells.

2. Fructose

Like glucose, fructose is also a *monosaccharide*, or single unit sugar. It is a "fruit sugar," common (not surprisingly) in fruit, but is also found in vegetables. Unlike glucose which immediately enters the bloodstream and raises blood sugar, fructose is processed primarily by the liver, and therefore has little immediate effect on blood sugar. This initially gave fructose a "healthy" label, when in fact fructose bears quite a few demons.

When processed in the liver, fructose promotes fat storage rather than oxidation. Once processed into fat by the liver, fructose is shipped out on proteins, raising triglyceride levels in the blood stream. Fructose also does not raise leptin levels which regulate satiety, so fructose does not quell the appetite. Fructose encourages the formation of advanced glycation end-products (AGEs) which accelerate aging. Fructose is linked to non-alcoholic fatty liver disease, pancreatic cancer, metabolic syndrome, and high cholesterol. Those particularly intolerant to fructose may also experience digestive issues such as gas and bloating.

3. Sucrose

Sucrose is a *disaccharide*, or combination of glucose and fructose in a 1:1 ratio. It is usually produced from refined sugar cane or sugar beets, and appears as white table sugar. Sucrose is highly inflammatory in nature, while its glucose/fructose combination renders it *especially* problematic.

Sucrose misleadingly registers lower on the glycemic index compared to glucose, but this is due to its fructose content, which minimally affects blood sugar in the short term. The presence of fructose, however, renders sucrose all the more dangerous. When you ingest sucrose (glucose + fructose), the glucose part enters the bloodstream, encouraging insulin release, while the fructose goes to the liver, further encouraging fat storage and advanced glycation end-products. Can you say bad combination?

4. Other Forms Of Sugar

Sugar also pops up in the form of *corn syrup, high fructose corn syrup (HFCS), honey, maple syrup, molasses, agave nectar,* as well as many others. I'll focus on HFCS (the premiere sweetener of processed foods and beverages) as well as honey and agave, since they are often categorized as potentially "Paleo" in nature.

High Fructose Corn Syrup (HFCS)

More than 40% of added caloric sweeteners in the US are in the form of high fructose corn syrup (HFCS), the premiere sweetener of processed foods and beverages (especially soft drinks). Americans on average consume around *60 pounds* of HFCS per year. While different versions exist, HFCS yields close to a 50/50 ratio of glucose and fructose, but in liquid form, making it essentially liquid sucrose.

Between 1970 and 1990, HFCS consumption increased more than 1000%, mirroring the rise of the obesity epidemic. Readily available to the body in liquid form, HFCS takes the glucose + fructose problem of sucrose and makes it much worse. To recap the glucose + fructose problem: the glucose part spikes blood sugar and insulin, while the fructose part promotes fat storage. HFCS is nefarious stuff, and is strongly correlated to the obesity epidemic, diabetes, and all the problems arising from such. In fact, rats with access to HFCS gain significantly more weight than those with access to sucrose, even when they consume *the same amount of calories*. Even more telling for the evils of HFCS, the sucrose consumed in the rat experiment was the equivalent "strength" of sugar found in soft drinks, while the HFCS was actually *watered down* from the common form.

Honey
Honey is probably the most natural "sugary" thing you can find in the wild. Like sucrose and HFCS, honey features fructose and glucose. Unlike refined sugar, honey contains minerals, amino acids, antioxidants and B vitamins. However, honey is comparable on the glycemic index to white table sugar - both are in the low to mid 60s, and is high in the nefarious fructose. If you're trying to eradicate your sweet tooth, honey probably won't help matters much. While many Paleo people consume honey, it's hard to justify any refined sort of sugar in the diet. I vote avoid honey, and get your nutrients and sweetness from whole food sources. There's nothing in honey you *can't* get from other whole foods, and without the insulin spike.

Agave
Agave nectar is a highly concentrated sweetener produced from the blue agave plant - a flowering plant which looks like a cactus. (It's also the same plant which gives us tequila. Oh hey!) Agave nectar can be up to *90% fructose,* which is substantially higher than high fructose corn syrup's 50%. This is really bad news. Fructose is metabolized primarily by the liver, promotes fat storage, fails to induce satiety, and can contribute to non-alcoholic fatty liver disease. Avoid agave. It's basically just refined liquid fructose. Your body doesn't care that it "was once a plant." Really.

A NOTE ON FRUIT AND VEGETABLE SUGAR

Fruits are quite high in sugar (especially fructose), as are starchy vegetables (featuring primarily glucose). While fruits are definitely healthy whole foods, many have been selectively bred to contain far more sugar than their ancestors. Furthermore, I find many people do not grasp the concept that *all carbs are sugar*, and so a completely fruit and vegetable based diet is a sugar based diet. This often comes up when discussing raw diets or juice cleanses. While I think such methods may be beneficial due to their inevitable calorie restriction, maximization of nutrient absorption, and minimization of toxins, such protocols are still a sugar-based diet. Even if you only drink green juices, that is still *a lot* of sugar, and sugar in large quantities just isn't ideal. When it comes to fruit and vegetables, favor their whole, natural form. Avoid refining them via dehydration or juicing.

CHAPTER FOUR

FAKE PROBLEMS

Similar to the plant anti-nutrient concept discussed in Chapter 2: *Grainy Problems*, processed foods also wreak havoc on the body. Although the chemicals, toxins, preservatives, and flavorings in processed foods may taste delicious, our body easily registers these compounds as foreign invaders, yielding an immune response, systemic inflammation, and state of self-attack.

FOOD ADDITIVES

Food additives overwhelmingly color today's plethora of boxed and canned goodies, both figuratively and literally. Figuratively, we've got *phenols, glycerin, MSG, sulfites,* and *carrageenan,* as well as cancer-promoting carcinogens such as *nitrates, nitrosamines, pesticides,* and *dioxins*. On the literal side, we've got *food dyes*, which actually affect the color of the intestines, to give you an idea of their potency. (I guess it's true how my mother always insisted Kool-Aid would *"turn your insides blue!"*) These unnatural chemicals and dyes place a toxic burden on the body, can negatively alter gut flora, and encourage allergies and autoimmune conditions.

TRANS FATS

Processed foods are often high in trans fats, which are artificially created unsaturated fats (although they may exist in minute amounts in animal fats). Trans fats are made by chemically tweaking hydrogen molecules to make the fat more shelf stable and heat resilient. See Chapter 5: *Fat Problems* for more on this.

Trans fats harm endothelial function, raise bad cholesterol, and lower good cholesterol. They are overwhelmingly linked to diabetes and heart disease (an accusation often erroneously placed upon saturated fat). Trans fats also increase blood levels of inflammatory biomarkers like C-reactive protein. In a study of 730 women, CRP levels were a whopping 73% higher in women consuming larger doses of trans fats. By creating systemic inflammation, trans fats can also encourage any of the autoimmune conditions previously discussed.

While trans fats are listed on food labels, a serving size can legally contain up to .5 grams and still be listed as zero. In products with small serving sizes (like in sauces), "zero" trans fats may actually add up quite quickly, and even smaller amounts may be harmful as well.

JUNK FOOD ADDICTION

Ever had that moment where you simply *had* to eat another one of those pre-packaged cookies or slice of suspiciously colorful sheet cake, even though you weren't really hungry or, in all honesty, it didn't even taste that amazing? Guess what! It's not all in your mind!

Well, it is… but that's the point.

Processed foods are highly addictive, and not in a casual "hard to resist" way. Actually, processed foods (hereafter referred to as "junk food") can be *literally* addictive. They're scientifically designed to be highly palatable and trigger the mesolimbic dopaminergic system, or "reward section," of our brain - the same neural circuits activated in drug or alcohol addiction.

In the healthily functioning body, a person's "appetite" adequately moderates energy intake and deficits, making you feel hungry when you *need* food, and full when you do not. Junk food disrupts this system by increasing hunger while simultaneously decreasing satiety signals (even though it "should" be doing the opposite, since junk food is typically high in calories). As noted in the 2011 *FASEB Journal*, "Activation of the mesolimbic reward pathway creates a sense of pleasure and interferes with physiological satiety signals, which promotes the further consumption of palatable foods."

In fact, rats given access to "cafeteria food" (i.e.: junk food) quickly develop binge eating habits. Other rodent studies show sucrose consumption instigates dopamine release in the brain. When rats are conditioned to associate sucrose with the cue of pushing a lever, they will eventually experience dopamine hits once they press the lever, even *before* the sucrose is actually delivered, and even if no sucrose is delivered at all.

Tying into our hedonistic pathways like an addictive drug such as cocaine or heroin, junk foods provide a "hit" of pleasure, while raising the threshold for that pleasure. More and more of the substance is then required to achieve the same effect. In clinical studies, rats fed diets of junk food would voluntarily undergo *painful shocks* in order to receive more of the junk food. As noted in 2010 *Nature Neuroscience,* "Overconsumption of palatable food triggers addiction-like neuroadaptive responses in brain reward circuitries and drives the development of compulsive eating." Those poor rats. And poor humans, as represented by the rats.

Alterations to the brain's neural network for appetite regulation from junk food can even begin in the womb. One study found that when pregnant rats were fed junk food, it altered the mesolimbic reward pathway of the offspring. The baby rats were more inclined to seek out highly palatable junk food and become obese. This is especially troublesome, given that, as of 2013, more than 50% of women are overweight or obese when pregnant. In other words, a majority of children born today may be "programmed" from the beginning to crave junk food.

Even though I've been low carb for more than half a decade, and Paleo for over 2 years, I *still* struggle when walking by any food product advertised by that deviously cuddlicious Pillsbury Doughboy, be it the crescent rolls, cinnamon rolls, slice and bake cookies, or Funfetti cake. The moment I pass such scrumptious temptations in the store, or even *think* about them, I am overwhelmed with insatiable gluttonous thoughts of *"I WANT IT NOW."* In fact, I must now cease writing for a moment, because the cravings are hitting me full force.

Melanie Avalon

{Moment to collect myself.}

The What When Wine Diet

And we're back! See, all it takes is a moment of sanity! Please rest assured that you are not alone in your cravings, which are thanks to *brilliant* food scientists and manufacturers screwing you over. But know you *can* resist. Though I've dreamt of it often, I haven't actually eaten any of that doughboy's goodies in years. Though I occasionally hanker for the neon sprinkled cake, I know even a minuscule taste will only make me want it *that much more*. Like any drug, just say no! Reflect on the rats shocking themselves. Not worth it.

Chapter Five

Fat Problems

The title here is a bit misleading, since the problem with dietary fat isn't so much that it's a problem; rather, it's a problem *that* it's a problem. If you follow me. Eating fat is *not* what makes you fat. At least not in the most basic sense. Nor is it unhealthy. Yet how often do I find myself at a restaurant, debating between the prime rib and filet mignon, when my salivations are interrupted by a friend's lament:

> *"Oh I want the steak, but I'll be good and get the low fat veggie pasta."*

Now back in my "Standard American Diet" (SAD) days, I'd eye my companion with a sort of envy, begrudging his or her self control, as I apparently had none. Now, however, I simply bite my tongue, eschew a soft sigh, and mumble something to the effect of, *"Get the steak. It's fine."* The dinner table is no place for a debate on food politics, even though politics have defined its current manifestation. Old habits die hard. Old dietary dogma based on myths? They may just be immortal.

THE DEFAMATION OF FAT

There's a very complicated and twisted history to the vilification of dietary fat. If you want the full story, consider reading *Good Calories, Bad Calories: Fats, Carbs, and the Controversial Science of Diet and Health* by Gary Taubes, or *The Big Fat Surprise: Why Butter, Meat and Cheese Belong in a Healthy Diet* by Nina Teicholz.

But I shall attempt a brief summary. History lesson time!

It all started in the 1950s, when a scientist by the name of Ancel Keys theorized that high amounts of saturated fat (a type of fat naturally found in animal products) increased cholesterol and thereby promoted heart disease. In support of this idea, he published an extensive "Seven Countries Study" showing that countries with diets low in saturated fat experienced less heart disease. In 1961, Keys achieved celebrity status by gracing the cover of *Time* magazine to proclaim the evils of saturated fat. The *American Heart Association*, a private company funded by *Procter & Gamble* (manufacturers of "Crisco," a notably soy-based fat) jumped on board. In 1977 the government joined the crusade, publishing its first *Dietary Goals for the United States*, which advocated increased carbohydrate intake and decreased fat intake for heart health – the first government publication regarding diet risk factors. The low fat diet for health mantra was born!

The problem? This *colossal* cultural shift was a vast assumption of medical advice based on inconclusive and skewed evidence. For starters, Keys' "Seven Countries Study" was uncontrolled and correlational, looking at broad trends easily involving a myriad of factors, rather than cause and effect data. More importantly, while Keys gathered data for 21 countries, he cherry picked 7 which supported his theory. Countries with high dietary fat but low heart disease were omitted, such as France, Germany, Holland, and Switzerland, as were those with low dietary fat but high levels of heart disease, like Chili. Contradictions were also dismissed, such as in Finland, where the Eastern side featured significantly more heart disease than the Western, despite *equivalent* fat intakes. If you pick 7 *different* countries from Keys' data, the saturated fat/heart disease link evanesces.

Problems also brewed in Keys' keystone (pun intended) country which supported his saturated fat/heart disease theory: the island of

Crete (which is the basis for the Mediterranean diet). Keys visited the island during an anomalous time in their diet history, when they suffered dietary hardship from World War II. The study was also conducted during Lent, effectively minimizing meat and cheese consumption. The low fat dietary data Keys collected from this island of low heart disease was therefore not representative of the country's normal, fattier diet.

Actual *controlled* studies of fat at the time in patient diets were overwhelmingly inconclusive, ultimately favoring no saturated fat/ heart disease connection. As Taubes notes, only two trials actually looked at a low fat diet's effect on heart disease (as opposed to a polyunsaturated vs. saturated fat diet's effect on heart disease). While one indicated a low fat diet reduced heart disease rates, the other indicated it did not. That means there were *two* studies in total addressing this exhalation of a low fat diet... and they contradicted each other.

As for the other studies on polyunsaturated fats *replacing* saturated fats in diet in relation to heart disease, the results were even less supportive. Some showed polyunsaturated fat diets reduced heart disease, but increased death rates overall (kind of defying the purpose). Others simply showed no correlation. In fact, a 2010 meta-analysis reviewing 21 studies on reduced saturated fat and cardiovascular health reported that "there is no significant evidence for concluding that dietary saturated fat is associated with an increased risk of CHD (coronary heart disease) or CVD (cardiovascular disease)."

And ironically, the government's *Dietary Goals* published in 1977 were on point spirit wise, crediting the increase in degenerative diseases to diet. As its preface noted, "Major health problems are diet related. Most all of the health problems underlying the leading causes of death in the United States could be modified by improvements in diet." Yet while the guidelines did advocate a lower sugar intake, they focused on decreasing fat intake and increasing carbohydrate intake. (Which, as we discussed in Chapter 3: *Sweet Problems*, indirectly increases sugar intake.) Why was fat demonized rather than sugar? Why did a "low fat" diet strike the nation, rather than a "low sugar" one?

As for the relationship between fats and cholesterol (Keys' original thesis), irony reigns, since dietary cholesterol minimally affects blood cholesterol levels. Cholesterol is a waxy lipid substance in the body with a myriad of purposes, including building cell membranes, assimilating vitamins, and synthesizing sex hormones. It is found in dietary fat. However, the cholesterol you eat does *not* automatically pop up in your blood stream. Unlike something else. {cough} Sugar. {cough} Furthermore, cholesterol is divided into two main types: *LDL* and *HDL*. In excess, LDL, or "bad cholesterol," can form plaque on artery walls, restricting blood flow and encouraging heart disease. HDL, or "good cholesterol," removes excess LDL from the bloodstream. While dietary saturated fats do slightly raise "bad" LDL cholesterol levels, they simultaneously raise "good" HDL cholesterol levels, which regulate the LDL cholesterol. This renders them essentially insignificant in regards to total cholesterol levels. Furthermore, there are different types of LDL: dangerous dense, sticky ones; and puffy, billowy particles which are more benign. Fats tend to raise the better billowy version of LDL, while carbs raise the dense, sticky "bad" version. (Perhaps it is sugar, not fat, which increases heart disease?) In fact, the one type of dietary fat which *does* specifically raise bad cholesterol and lower good cholesterol is *trans fat*, a type of fat overwhelmingly generated in commercial products, in response to the demonization of saturated fat. *(Oh hey low fat margarine!)* Such irony.

Despite the utter lack of scientific evidence to reduce fat intake in the 1950s-70s, Americans were in a prime position to accept any heart disease theory offered, as officials proclaimed heart disease strikingly on the rise. In actuality, this "rise" was likely due to a myriad of factors, such as the decline of deaths from infectious diseases (thanks to modern medicine), which left older humans susceptible to degenerative diseases like heart disease and cancer. The year 1949 also saw the addition of "arteriosoclerotic heart disease" as a category on death certificates. After its inclusion, heart disease rates "rose" by 20-35% within the year, since it could now be cited as a cause of death. Furthermore, the *1948 National Heart Act* and creation of the *National Heart Institute* supported a substantial influx of government funding into heart disease awareness and prevention, beginning with an unprecedented $9 million for heart research. President Eisenhower's heart attack in 1955 sealed the deal for the new fearful heart ethos.

Perhaps most importantly, the *American Heart Association*, a private institution funded by the aforementioned "Crisco" sponsors, while initially skeptical of the sketchy science behind the attack on fat, ultimately chose to embrace the anti-fat movement clearly so in vogue. In 1957, the AHA dismissed Keys' theories as faulty, with insubstantial evidence. In 1960, *despite no change in the evidence,* the AHA adamantly proclaimed that "the best scientific evidence of the time" called for low fat intakes for heart health.

And so, advised to lower fat intake at all costs, despite a lack of legitimately supportive evidence, Americans eagerly turned to high carb, low fat diets featuring grains, sugar, and processed foods. Food manufacturers jumped on board by churning out polyunsaturated margarines to replace butter, and "healthy" low fat, fake fats. (I cringe just writing this.)

The damage was done. Heart disease rates continued to rise. Oh, and we got the obesity epidemic and diabetes influx as a bonus! So next time you choose that salad with low fat dressing instead of the steak, and decline the butter, you can know that politics have done their job at the dinner table. If by doing their job, we mean potentially ruining your health while instigating a less satisfying eating experience to boot.

WHY YOU NEED FAT

Unlike carbs, you actually *need* fat. Yes, the stuff is actually *good* for you. Shocker. (I say that in jest, yet I know many, if not most, *do* find that shocking.) While both carbs and fats can be used as energy for the body, fats provide essential nutritional building blocks. To give you an idea, just consider that 50% of cell membranes are composed of fat, and 70% of the brain is fat. Fat is also vital for vitamin assimilation. The fat soluble vitamins A, D, E, and K are all stored in fat.

Even more important, the *"essential fatty acids"* (EFAs) *alpha-linolenic* and *linoleic acid* must be obtained from food. These include the well-known Omega-3 and Omega-6s. Protein is also essential. What about the "essential" carbs, you ask? There are none. The minute amount of glucose required by the body is easily satisfied by a low carb diet. But even if you ate *no* carbs, the body can generate glucose from fat and protein. I did this for a good 6 months or so my last year of college. My neighborhood grocery store would mark down the rotisserie chickens to $3 each night, so I just ate an *entire* chicken with coconut oil every night. It was a pretty fantastic, albeit pre-Paleo, passing phase. I now favor much more diversity and less additives, thank goodness.

FAT DOES NOT MAKE YOU FAT

Here's the thing. Eating fat is *not* what ultimately makes you fat. At least not in the most basic sense. Yes, our body stores excess calories in the form of fat. Those excess calories, however, can just as easily come from carbs (as they *typically* do). But even more importantly, *what* you eat determines the body's readiness for such storage. Eating fats do not "tell" your body to store fat. Carbs do that! Carbs "switch on" *insulin:* the hormone responsible for fat storage. When you eat carbs, you're telling your body to store fat. In such a situation, whatever dietary fat you *do* eat is merely along for the ride, and will more likely be stored as body fat. Dietary fat, however, *does not* raise insulin in and of itself, so while eating fat on a high carb diet will be easily stored, fat consumed on a low carb diet is *not* readily stored. On the contrary, it controls appetite and further encourages the body to burn dietary and body fat as fuel.

DIFFERENT TYPES OF FAT

So what exactly *is* fat? Fats are composed of carbon, hydrogen, and oxygen atoms. The amount of hydrogen atoms present determines the amount of "bonds" existing between the carbon atoms. The amount of bonds between the carbons determines the "type" of fat. Stick with me here. (Pun intended.)

There are two parent categories of fats: *saturated* and *unsaturated*. In *saturated fats,* all the carbons are fully "saturated" by hydrogen atoms, so each carbon is only connected to each other by a single bond. *Unsaturated fats,* on the other hand, feature less hydrogen atoms, which the carbons "make up for" by creating double bonds with fellow carbons. One double bond creates a *monounsaturated fat,* while multiple double bonds create a *polyunsaturated fat.* The more carbon double bonds, the more fluid the fat. (Think of the bonds as being "bendy" places in the fat chain.) These double bonds are less stable and easily react with oxygen, or "oxidize." In other words, they easily go rancid.

Note: While people often categorize dietary fats as a single type (i.e.: animal fat is "saturated" and olive oil is "monounsaturated"), most foods typically feature multiple types of fat.

1. Saturated Fats

Saturated fats are found mostly in butter and animal fats. They contain no double bonds: all the carbons in the fatty acids are "saturated" in hydrogen atoms. They are solid at room temperature and very stable. You don't have to worry so much about them spoiling or oxidizing, including in your body. Saturated fats contain fat soluble vitamins like K, A, and D. They make up 50% of the body's cell membranes, and support calcium, vitamin, and essential fatty acid synthesis. While saturated fats do elevate cholesterol, they raise both HDL and LDL, rendering them benign in the grand scheme of things.

Furthermore, a short chain saturated fatty acid called *butyrate* (found abundantly in grass-fed ghee and butter) is actually anti-inflammatory in nature. It has been shown in scientific studies to suppress pro-inflammatory cytokines and support a healthy gut homeostasis. In fact, the good gut bacteria convert soluble fibers into butyrate, which then serves as an energy source for the colon. If you want to remember this awesome fatty acid and how to integrate it into your diet, just remember that **but**yrate gets its name from **but**ter. Oh hey!

2. Monounsaturated Fats

Monounsaturated fats are found in many nut, seed, and fruit oils, like olive, sesame seed, and safflower oil. Interestingly, they also constitute a good percentage of animal fat as well. About 30% of butter and almost half of lard (AKA bacon fat!) is monounsaturated fat. Monounsaturated fats contain one "double bond" between fatty acids and are typically liquid at room temperature, but may gel or solidify when cooled. While not as stable as saturated fats, monounsaturated fats don't go rancid as easily as polyunsaturated fats. They are a nice alternative to trans fats and the inflammatory Omega-6 polyunsaturated fats (see below) which define our modern diet. Monounsaturated fats may support good cholesterol levels, and reduce risk of breast cancer, heart disease, and stroke.

I've found that monounsaturated fats tend to get ignored in the Paleo sphere, a community often focused on defending saturated fat and highlighting the damage done by Omega-6 polyunsaturated fats. As such, monounsaturated fats often fall by the wayside. They're healthy. Eat them!

3. Polyunsaturated Fats

Polyunsaturated fats are abundant in fish, nuts, and grains. As such, they constitute a huge percent of the modern diet. They contain more than one double bond between fatty acids. They're pretty much always liquid, and easily oxidize (or go rancid). Polyunsaturated fats are a double-edged sword in that they can be both super awesome, yet super damaging. It all goes back to those ever famous Omega-3 and Omega-6 fatty acids. Allow me to explain.

Essential Fatty Acids (EFAs)

There are two specific types of polyunsaturated fats required by the body, which the body cannot synthesize on its own. You must get them from the food you eat, no way around it. These are *linoleic acid (LA)* found in the polyunsaturated *Omega-6s*, and *alpha-linolenic acid (ALA)* found in *Omega-3s*. While both are required, Omega-6s are inflammatory, while Omega-3s are anti-inflammatory. Let's say that again! Omega-6s are inflammatory, while Omega-3s are anti-inflammatory. One more time! Omega-6s are inflammatory, while Omega-3s are anti-inflammatory.

Omega-6s are abundant in processed seed and vegetable oils (like corn, peanut, and soybean), while Omega-3s are found in flaxseed, walnuts, and fatty fish (particularly salmon, herring, sardines, and oysters). Conventional meats contain more Omega-6s, while grass-fed meats feature more Omega-3s.

EFAs make up cell membranes throughout the body, from immune cells, to red blood cells, to cardiac and neural tissue. They affect the cells' flexibility, fluidity, and activity. They're pretty important stuff! EFA deficiency can lead to skin rashes, stunted growth, dampened immune system, vision problems, and declined cognitive functioning.

The Omega-6:3 Ratio

Historically, we consumed Omega-6 and Omega-3s in a 1:1 ratio, maximizing benefits and discouraging negative effects. Our modern processed diet rampant in grains and vegetable oils, however, yields an estimated *16:1* Omega-6:3 ratio. Scary stuff. Since the cells of our body are *literally* made of these essential fatty acids from diet, a skewed Omega-6:3 ratio causes a shift towards a cellular foundation of inflammation. This encourages every inflammatory problem you can imagine, from cardiovascular problems, to autoimmune diseases, to cancer. Omega-3s, on the other hand, are anti-inflammatory and protective against such conditions. Studies show they decrease cardiovascular diseases, diabetes, and mortality rates in general. They may help with inflammatory conditions such as rheumatoid arthritis and inflammatory bowel disease (IBS). Omega-3 deficiencies may even play a part in the development of psychiatric disorders such as bipolar disorder and depression. In fact, pregnant women may experience postpartum depression (characterized by sleep difficulties, crying, fatigue, and loss of appetite) because the fetus utilizes his or her mother's Omega-3 fatty acids for developing brain and nervous tissue.

It is prudent to maximize Omega-3 intake, while minimizing Omega-6 intake. The ratio is so "off" in today's diet, that you really don't have to worry about underconsuming Omega-6s or overconsuming Omega-3s.

EPA & DHA

While most Omega-3s (the good stuff!) consumed in today's diet are the aforementioned *ALA* (alpha-linolenic acid) from vegetarian sources like flaxseed and walnuts, the specific type of Omega-3 found in *fatty fish* is actually the long chain *EPA* (eicosapentaenoic acid) and *DHA* (docosahexaenoic acid). EPA and DHA provide *more potent health benefits* than ALA. Although ALA from vegetarian sources can be converted to EPA and DHA, the conversion is costly. Therefore, consuming Omega-3s from fatty fish is the ideal route to follow. Women are notably more efficient at converting ALA into DHA and EPA than men, and thus may benefit even more from Omega-3 fish supplementation (since their body clearly favors it). DHA is particularly important for vision and brain function, with studies linking DHA deficiencies to learning deficits. It is also critical for infant development. In fact, women preferentially store DHA in their thigh fat, which is reserved for pregnancy to nurture the child. (See Chapter 18: *Fat Burning, IF Style* for more on that.)

If all of that was confusing, here's a quick recap! Polyunsaturated fats are the most liquid fats and easily spoil. They contain the only actual essential fats which *must* be consumed through diet, called EFAs. These EFAs are Omega-6 and Omega-3. Omega-6 is inflammatory, while Omega-3 is anti-inflammatory. Today we eat *way too much* Omega-6, and therefore should focus on *minimizing Omega-6 intake while adding more Omega-3s*. As for Omega-3s, they come in the form of ALA in flaxseed and walnuts, and EPA and DHA in fatty fish. EPA and DHA are the best form of Omega-3 for health. If you take away nothing else from this section, know that eating fatty fish is awesome for your health!

4. Medium Chain Triglycerides (MCTs)

Medium Chain Triglycerides are a type of saturated fat found primarily in coconut and palm oil. They're the darling of the Paleo world, with a stunning list of benefits. Unlike the other saturated and unsaturated fats which must be broken down in the intestines to be used as energy and stored as fats, MCTs are sent directly to the liver for energy. As such, they act similar to carbohydrates in providing instant fuel, yet without the insulin spike! MCTs also encourage *ketone* production, an energy substrate supporting the body in general, but particularly the brain. MCTs can discourage fat gain, decrease appetite, upregulate fatty acid use, enhance thermogenesis, and regulate insulin. They support the immune system and absorption of calcium and magnesium. They can act as antioxidants, reduce cholesterol, and protect against a myriad of diseases, such as cirrhosis, pancreatitis, Crohn's disease, and malabsorption in newborns.

Plus coconut oil just tastes delicious! You can add it to salads, veggies, or meats, or even eat it plain! Buy the virgin, unrefined version. I like the *Trader Joe's* and *Whole Foods* store brands of unrefined coconut oil. They're both relatively inexpensive as well.

5. Trans Fats

Trans fats are bad news all around. These are chemically modified fats in which normally liquid vegetable fats are "hydrogenated," meaning their hydrogen atoms are tweaked in order to make the fat more solid and shelf stable. Since they can withstand high temperatures, trans fats are often used in the food industry for frying. They're also resistant to spoilage, and thus are abundant in processed foods, baked goods, and "low fat" or "fake fat" foods like margarine.

The problem? Trans fats are just *really bad for you*, basically enacting all the bad stuff that saturated fats were "supposed" to do. They raise bad cholesterol and lower good cholesterol. They encourage inflammation and insulin resistance. And unlike saturated fats, they actually *do* increase risks of heart disease and diabetes.

Thankfully, a Paleo diet effectively frees you from these sneaky devils, so you shouldn't have to worry about them!

SO WHAT DOES IT ALL MEAN?

I know there's quite a lot to take in regarding fats, so here's the takeaway: *fats are a vital and healthy macronutrient not to be feared.* Save any such trepidation for sugar! The presence of carbs in one's diet rather than fat is what ultimately determines the body's preference for fat storage, and the myriad of degenerative diseases arising from such. Fat intake is really only problematic in the form of trans fats, excess Omega-6s, or on a high carb diet (since such a condition encourages their ultimate storage rather than use).

For practical application, try to get your fat from whole food sources (like meat and avocado) rather than slathering foods in oil. If you can afford it, favor grass-fed over conventional meats to idealize Omega-6:3 ratios. If you can't afford it, choose leaner cuts. Either way, eat fatty fish and supplement with Omega-3s via fish oil. Avoid trans fats at all costs, minimize vegetable oils, but embrace MCTS, commonly found in coconut oil. And most importantly, do not fear fat! As long as sugar is avoided, fat = health!

Chapter Six

How To Do Paleo

If you thought we'd never get here... here we are! (Unless of course you jumped straight to this chapter without all the backstory, which would be a regrettable, yet understandable approach. To each his own.)

A Paleo diet embraces an abundance of hearty, delicious whole foods, while eliminating inflammatory grains, processed and refined foods, and added sugars. Think natural. If it's an animal, then it's Paleo. If it's a plant or vegetable naturally existing in the wild, and you can walk up and eat it without any problem, then it's Paleo. Otherwise... it's probably not Paleo. If it contains unpronounceable ingredients sounding like they came from a lab... also probably not Paleo.

PALEO YES LIST
Eat these foods as much as you want, and to satiety! Paleo-friendly foods high in carbohydrates are noted with a *, and should be avoided if you choose a lower carb Paleo approach. **The examples under each category are not exhaustive.**

Meat
Beef
Bison
Chicken
Duck
Goat
Lamb
Pork
Seafood: *Fish, Lobster, Shrimp, etc.*
Turkey
Veal

Vegetables
Artichoke
Asparagus
Avocado
Beets*
Broccoli
Brussels Sprouts
Cabbage
Carrot*
Cauliflower
Cucumber
Celery
Kale
Lettuce
Mushroom
Onion
Radish
Spinach
Squash*
Sweet Potato*
Turnip
Yam*

Fruits
- Apple
- Banana*
- Blackberry
- Blueberry
- Cherry*
- Fig*
- Grape*
- Grapefruit
- Lemon
- Lime
- Oranges*
- Peach*
- Pineapple*
- Plums*
- Raspberry
- Strawberry
- Watermelon*

Nuts & Seeds
- Almond
- Cashew
- Coconut
- Hazelnut
- Macadamia
- Pecan
- Pine Nuts
- Pistachio
- Walnut

Natural Oils/Fats
- Avocado Oil
- Coconut Oil
- Flaxseed Oil
- Olive Oil
- Palm Oil
- Ghee

PALEO NO LIST
Avoid these like the plague!

Grains
Barley
Cereals
Corn
Oats
Rice
Wheat

Legumes
Beans - *Black, Green, String, Lima, etc.*
Lentils
Miso
Peas - *Black-eyed, Chick, English, etc.*
Peanuts, Peanut Butter
Soybeans, Tofu

Added/Refined Sugars
Agave
Coconut Sugar
Dextrose
Sucrose
Fructose

Refined/Hydrogenated/Processed Oils
Canola Oil
Soybean Oil
Vegetable Oil

Anything Packaged/Processed
Most Boxed Foods, Snacks, Condiments, etc.
Processed Meats - *Hot Dogs, Deli Meats, etc.*
Artificial Colors, Flavors, Preservatives
Aspartame
GMOs
MSG (monosodium glutamate)
Nitrates
Saccharin
Sucralose

PALEO MAYBE LIST

The following foods are typically discouraged in the Paleo diet, and should definitely be avoided during the initial 30 days or so, but may be reintroduced and sustained if they do not cause problems. See Chapter 11: *Paleo Q&A* for elaboration.

Dairy (*favor grass-fed and raw varieties*)
- Butter
- Cheese
- Cream Cheese
- Egg
- Ice Cream
- Milk
- Yogurt

Nightshades
- Goji Berries
- Peppers
- Potatoes
- Tomatoes
- Zucchini

Alcohol
- Clear Liquors - *Vodka, Gin, Tequila, etc.*
- Wine

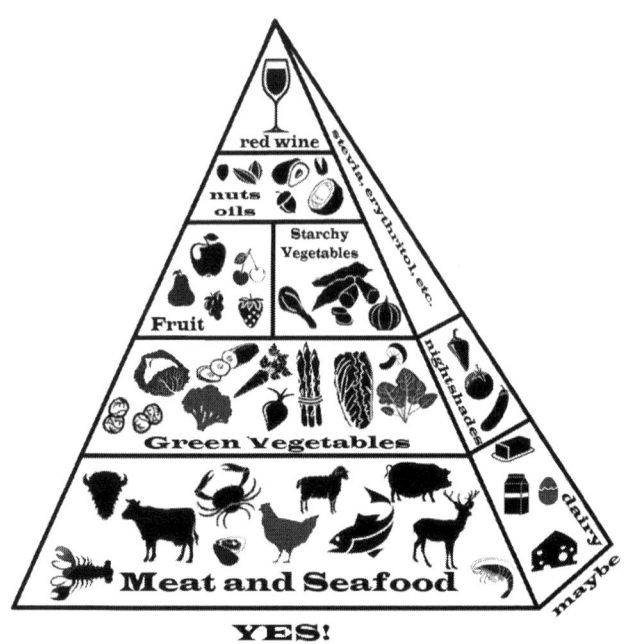

PALEO PYRAMID

HOW TO START PALEO

I believe jumping all in is the best and ultimately easiest approach to starting Paleo, at least in retrospect. True adherence is the quickest way to eliminate cravings, which often linger when you keep them present via chemical substitutes or cheat meals. It's like seeing your ex-boyfriend or ex-girlfriend everyday, compared to moving to a different state and never seeing them again. Which situation is easier for moving on? Furthermore, an extended period of strict adherence is vital for complete elimination of inflammatory and allergenic foods, as even seemingly small exposures can ignite damage and inflammation.

Both Robb Wolf's *The Paleo Solution* (http://robbwolf.com) and Dallas and Melissa Hartwig's *Whole 30* program (http://www.whole30.com) advocate 100% strict adherence to the Paleo protocol for 30 days. I recommend this approach as well. After 30 days, you can individually reintroduce questionable "maybe" foods like dairy, nightshades, and alcohol, to see if they cause problems for you personally. They may or may not - individual tolerances vary.

Once you begin experiencing the increased energy, health, and vitality (not to mention weight loss!), Paleo quickly becomes a breeze. Cravings for toxic and sugary foods vanish, and you begin desiring just the good stuff! I now crave vegetables, which I used to disdain. True story. I cannot advocate complete commitment enough, and therefore suggest the 30 day trial run.

With all that said, while I *want* to say *"You must commit 100%!"* I know people function differently, and you've got to do what works for *you* personally. Although I can promise and proclaim that you'll feel substantially better with complete adherence, and that Paleo will become effortless soon (as it will), if such an idea is *inconceivable!* to you, then by all means, take it slow.

I must remember that my own transition to Paleo was a slow one. I adopted low carb (Atkins) long before Paleo, and used quite a few nefarious low carb chemical substitutes for both sugar and flour. Granted, I eventually weaned myself off them after adjusting to the lack of grains and sugar, but in retrospect, skipping the in-between stage would have made the transition much easier. Substitutions and cheats simply sustain cravings, allowing non-Paleo foods to hold a tempting power over you, and the goal here is to nip that temptation in the bud!

CHAPTER SEVEN

TRANSITIONING TO PALEO

If the *all-in 30 days approach* to Paleo is simply too much for you to handle, consider the following alternatives:

> 1. Start by eliminating just sugar, and then grains (or vice versa).
>
> 2. If you cannot commit to a month, try at least 2 weeks. You can do anything for 2 weeks!
>
> 3. Substitute with Paleo-friendly and, worst case scenario, sort-of-Paleo-friendly alternatives for cravings.

SUBSTITUTION

If substitution is your thing, here are some common (and not-so-common) Paleo alternatives to satisfy sugar and grain cravings. I have divided them into the "strict" (which are actually Paleo) and "loose" (which are not quite Paleo). I've also noted ones to avoid altogether. When in doubt, err on the side of whole foods which *replace* previous addictions, rather than "Paleo-friendly" ingredients which *mimic* previous addictions.

Note: The *glycemic index* (GI) measures the extent to which a type of carbohydrate raises blood sugar, and is thus a good barometer for gauging different types of carbs. It is based on a scale of 100, with 100 being pure glucose. Low GI foods measure 1-55. Moderate GI foods measure 56–69. High GI foods measure 70-100. The glycemic index does not account for insulin production from other means.

GRAIN ALTERNATIVES
THE STRICT

1. Yams & Sweet Potatoes
Starchy Paleo-approved vegetables like yams and sweet potatoes can easily satisfy starchy and starchy-sweet cravings.

2. Squash
Spaghetti squash is a fantastic substitute for spaghetti, while zucchini is great for "pasta" in general. Pumpkin is fabulous for dessert recipes.

3. Cauliflower
Mashed up cauliflower (try a food processor) can make excellent "mashed potatoes," especially with some grass-fed butter or bacon. Cauliflower can also serve as a rice substitute.

4. Cabbage
Try grilling cabbage in coconut oil for a nice chip replacement! Sautéed cabbage can also add a nice bulk to dishes, if you miss munching on high volume pasta, potatoes, etc.

5. Eggplant
While being a nightshade places it on the "Maybe" Paleo list, eggplant is pretty awesome in that it assumes any flavor with which it is cooked. It also adds nice substance to the meal.

THE LOOSE

1. Nut Flours
While not technically Paleo from the ancestral view given their refined nature, almond flour and coconut flour make great substitutes for baking. Be warned: it's easy to fall into the "mimic" habit, and go crazy with baked Paleo goodies. Tread carefully.

2. Shirataki Noodles
In my pre-Paleo, low carb days, I went through a Shirataki noodle phase (specifically a brand called "Miracle Noodle"). Made from the indigestible glucomannan fiber of the Konjac plant, shirataki noodles are tasteless, but assume the flavor of the ingredients with which they're cooked. They're a bit chewier than normal pasta, but can get the job done. I kind of shudder thinking about them now, since they're essentially massive amounts of indigestible fiber. However, you may fancy them, especially in the transition period. Make sure to always view the ingredient list, as many shirataki noodles are made with a soy blend.

3. Quinoa
Quinoa is a "pseudocereal" resembling grains and cereals, but is actually a seed more closely related to spinach. On the plus side, quinoa is a gluten-free "complete protein" providing all 9 essential amino acids. However, quinoa is carb intensive and quite high on the glycemic index at a 53 - slighter higher than wheat kernels, rice, and spaghetti. While some people tolerate it fine, quinoa does contains *saponins*, defensive compounds which may instigate digestive distress and intestinal permeability. I suggest avoiding quinoa in the beginning, then trying it later down the road if desired to see how you react.

AVOID

1. Soy
Both lauded and criticized, soy sparks constant debate. Like gluten, soy lurks everywhere. A 2003 report found soy present in more than 60% of processed foods, thanks to *textured soy protein* (a meat substitute and protein fortifier) and *soy protein isolate* (a protein enhancement). Processed forms of

soy such as tofu, soy milk, and tempeh, are typically full of unnecessary toxic additives. And in its natural form, the soybean is a *legume*, harboring toxic anti-nutrients like lectins, phytates, and saponins. (Although ironically, saponins are what bestow soy with its heralded "anti-cholesterol" property.)

The most complicated thing about soy, making it both potentially beneficial and harmful, is its high *phytoestrogen content*. Soy contains over 100 phytoestrogens: plant-derived hormone-like compounds which mimic estrogen in the body. As such, soy can increase or decrease estrogen levels. Benefits of this could include decreased menopausal symptoms and decreased risk of osteoporosis, as estrogen aids bone density retention. However, soy can negatively affect estrogen levels, leading to menstrual cycle delays, suppressed thyroid function, and breast cancer. Soy used in infant formulas is particularly problematic. As noted in *Frontiers in Neuroendocrinology,* "Manipulation of estrogen during specific critical windows of development throughout gestation and early infancy leads to a myriad of adverse health outcomes including malformations in the ovary, uterus, mammary gland and prostate, early puberty, reduced fertility, disrupted brain organization, and reproductive tract cancers."

While the soy craze has likely done much more harm than good, some people tolerate soybeans with minimal side effects. If you can do edamame and be ok, then by all means, do that edamame! But definitely avoid the generic processed soy stuff.

SUGAR ALTERNATIVES
THE STRICT
1. Fruit

Whole foods are the healthiest method to satisfy your sweet tooth. The most Paleo-friendly fruits are high in nutrients and antioxidants, while low in sugar. Consider berries (like raspberries, cranberries, blueberries, and blackberries), apples, pears, and grapefruit. Avoid high glycemic index fruits such as melons and bananas, as well as refined versions of fruits such as dried fruit or fruit juices.

THE LOOSE
1. Honey
Honey is probably the most natural "sugary" thing you can find in nature, containing fructose and glucose. Unlike refined sugar, honey contains minerals, amino acids, antioxidants, and B vitamins. However, honey is comparable on the glycemic index to white table sugar - both are in the low to mid 60s. If you're trying to get rid of your sweet tooth, honey won't help matters very much. Any refined sugar is bad news, increasing inflammation, glycation, fat storage, and insulin resistance.

AVOID
1. Agave Nectar
Agave nectar is a highly concentrated sweetener produced from the blue agave plant - a flowering plant which also gives us tequila. Agave nectar can be up to 90% fructose, which is substantially higher than High Fructose Corn Syrup's approximately 50%. Fructose is metabolized primarily by the liver, promotes fat storage, and can contribute to non-alcoholic fatty liver disease. Avoid agave. It's basically just liquid fructose.

ARTIFICIAL SWEETENERS
Artificial sweeteners are a tricky business. I went through quite the obsessive period myself. They're often demonized as cancer-causing packets of death, which is what I expected to find when researching them. However, as much as I hate to say it, low doses of artificial sweeteners *appear* to be relatively benign, at least from extreme cancer-producing viewpoints. They also do not raise blood sugar in general. That being said, I do believe artificial chemical sweeteners sustain our cravings for sweetness, mimic old habits, and are definitely "anti-Paleo" in spirit. Once I finally cut them out, I was much happier, and my Raynaud's syndrome finally went away. Recent studies are also implicating artificial sweeteners negatively affect the gut microbiome. I personally believe they may in fact wreck havoc on our gut bacteria, which are intimately tied to our overall health and immune system. I look forward to future research on the subject.

However, if you must sweeten something, I think some sugar

substitutes may be better than sugar. Stevia, for example, actually seems to provide some health benefits. (*SweetLeaf* is my favorite brand.) Sugar alcohols, especially erythritol, also seem relatively benign unless you have digestive problems.

Note: I reserve the right to take back everything I'm saying about these guys if future studies reveal more deleterious information on the subject. It really is tricky waters, so I cannot emphasize enough the importance of choosing whole foods over sweeteners.

TYPES OF ARTIFICIAL SWEETENERS

1. Saccharin (*Sweet'N Low* - the "pink packet")
Chemically derived from petroleum, Saccharin is the oldest "artificial sweetener," in use since the late 1800s. Saccharin is 300x sweeter than table sugar, and is not metabolized by the body, passing through unchanged. Although it suffered a backlash in the 1970s due to animal studies insinuating a connection to cancer, they have since been challenged and essentially dismissed. Recent rodent studies, however, have implicated that saccharin specifically may negatively affect the gut microbiome, inducing glucose intolerance (and who knows what else!) Further research is definitely needed.

2. Sucralose (*Splenda* - the "yellow packet")
Sucralose is actually a chemical modification of a sugar (sucrose) molecule, in which three hydrogen-oxygen groups are replaced with three chlorine atoms. It is 600x sweeter than sugar, and not metabolized by the body. Recent studies are showing sucralose may negatively affect the gut microbiome.

3. Aspartame (*Equal* - the "blue packet")
First created in 1965, Aspartame is about 200x sweeter than table sugar. Unlike the non-metabolized sucralose and saccharin, aspartame actually *is* broken down by the body into amino acids and methanol. Some worry about the methanol, but studies have shown no negative side effects up to 4000mg/kg of bodyweight per day. That being said, aspartame is probably the artificial sweetener to "most" avoid, since it is processed by the body. Recent studies are showing aspartame may negatively affect the gut microbiome.

4. Sugar Alcohols
Common sugar alcohols include *sorbitol, malitol, xylitol,* and *erythritol.* They contain around 6% of the calories of table sugar, but 50-70% of the sweetness, and taste similar. Their low glycemic indexes of 1-7 mean they negligibly affect blood sugar, and are considered safe for diabetics. They also may protect the teeth from cavities, which is a nice side benefit. Sugar alcohols are kind of like a combination between sugar and alcohol, and are difficult for the body to digest. High sugar alcohol intake may yield stomach upset and a laxative effect, due to poor processing by the body. While not ideal, sugar alcohols may be better than the previously discussed artificial sweeteners on the market.

5. Stevia
Stevia *might* just be the one processed sweetener that's dandy all around. The stevia sweetener comes from a South American herb plant of the same name, with extracts stevioside and rebaudioside which are about 250-300x sweeter than table sugar, but with an impressive GI of 0. This kind of makes stevia a winner, although some perceive a bitter aftertaste.

Unlike other processed sweeteners, stevia may actually have a few health benefits. Studies have shown stevia can help control blood sugar and insulin spikes after meals, and may help with hypertension. Furthermore, levels of satiety rate similar to sucrose. Look for stevia without additional additives. I've found *SweetLeaf* to be a safe brand with no aftertaste, in my opinion. The powdered form uses the benign inulin soluble fiber as its binding agent, while the liquid drops often just contain stevia and water. (Of course, always double check the ingredient list!)

Chapter Eight

Shopping, Paleo Style

Grocery shopping Paleo-style doesn't have to be difficult! While Paleo may seem expensive upfront, consider *nutrition versus dollar*. Packaged grains and processed foods may *seem* cheaper than meat and veggies, but if you look at the nutritional breakdown, you'll soon realize you're getting a lot more nutrition with whole foods. Here are some tips to help you save money and navigate the store, Paleo-style!

1. Buy In Bulk
Shop at places like Costco to buy wholesale - you can always freeze meat for months in the freezer. Products like oils can also be cheaper in the long run if you buy larger portions up front.

1. Broaden Your Horizons
When you go Paleo, you'll soon find you may like different cuts and types of meat than before. You don't have to stick to sirloins and chicken! I like to buy whatever cut of meat is on sale that week. Even tougher cuts of meat can be tasty

(and a crockpot can do wonders!) Also consider other types of meat, such as lamb or bison. Organ meats such as liver are also amazing for you, if you develop a taste for them! Think unconventionally when it comes to meals. Who says breakfast has to be pancakes? You can totally do meat and veggies for breakfast, or even dinner leftovers!

3. Frozen Foods
Frozen meats and veggies are often cheaper. Just make sure you check the ingredients for additives. Unlike canned vegetables, which often lose some of their nutrients in the canning process, frozen vegetables can be quite fresh. They can even be "fresher" than fresh vegetables, since they're frozen at their peak nutritional state (in theory), while the later are typically picked prematurely to allow ripening time in transport. Actual fresh vegetables are also more prone to spoilage.

Here are applicable meat storage times:

> **Poultry, raw:** 2 days fridge, 9 months freezer
> **Poultry, cooked:** 4 days fridge, 4 months freezer
> **Beef, raw:** 5 days fridge, 12 months freezer
> **Beef, cooked:** 4 days fridge, 3 months freezer
> **Meat, ground:** 2 days fridge, 4 months freezer
> **Fish, fresh:** 1 day fridge, 8 months freezer
> **Fish, cooked:** N/A fridge, 3 months freezer

4. Canned Foods
While not ideal because of potential metal toxicity, you can always stock up on canned meats and vegetables. I find this particularly helpful with salmon and other fish.

5. Choose Stores Wisely
When it comes to Paleo, I like more "natural" stores because they typically have more choices. I also feel more "at home" and less weird about my cart contents at such locales. *Trader Joe's* features natural products at awesome prices. I also love *Fresh & Easy,* which is fresh yet cheap, thanks to reduced staff from self-checkouts, and produce and meats with more pressing expiration dates. While *Whole Foods* basically has

every Paleo item you could want (*Oh hey 10 different types of raw sauerkraut!*), it can be a bit on the pricey side. Of course, you can still get food at your local *Kroger, Ralphs, Publix,* or other large chain - just be careful and read labels. Thankfully, even these stores are beginning to embrace the whole foods trend, featuring increasingly more Paleo-friendly "natural" and gluten-free foods.

6. Farmers Markets
You can get some pretty amazing, fresh food for good prices at local farmers markets! Don't be scared to ask questions and barter. Also consider going near the end of the day, when the farmers may be more inclined to lower prices. See the outing as a fun adventure with friends, rather than a grocery shopping trip!

7. Choose Organic Wisely
Don't stress too much about the whole organic/grass-fed thing at the beginning. The simple switch to whole foods will be an amazing step towards health and vitality, even with conventional foods. And when you do embrace the organic route (yey!), make smart choices.

For *produce*, the biggest concern is pesticides. Upgrade to organic for fruits and vegetables with a lot of edible surface area easily coated in toxins (such as leafy greens, apples, and strawberries). An avocado, for instance, probably doesn't need to be organic since the edible portion is on the inside. Consult the *Environmental Working Group* for a list of produce pesticide rates: http://www.ewg.org/foodnews/list.php. Even if you don't intend on buying organic, still check the organic prices. They *could* be on sale. It happens!

For *meat*, toxins accumulate in fat, so favor organic and grass-fed with the fattier cuts. If you're buying conventional chicken, consider buying it super lean, and then adding healthy fats like avocado, grass-fed butter, ghee, or coconut oil. If you have to decide between investing in organic produce versus organic meat, choose the meat. It is the foundation of the diet, after all!

8. Use Oils
Oils provide a lot of bang for their buck, calorie wise. Think

about how much energy is stored in a single jar of coconut or olive oil! You can easily make meals more tasty and satiating by adding them to your meats and salads.

9. Use Spices
Spices are cheap and nutritious, letting you easily prepare one type of meat many different ways, especially when used in junction with oils. Many spices also boast different health benefits. Turmeric, for example, is a wonder spice with anti-inflammatory properties, as is ginger, which also aids digestion.

10. Buy Online
You can buy things like oils and supplements online, often with free shipping if you have Amazon Prime! Amazon also has a "Subscribe and Save" option for slightly cheaper grocery-type items.

TRANSLATING FOOD LABELS

In the ideal modern world, we would be eating organic, natural, grass-fed, cage-free, free-range food all around, with such labels meaning what they imply. (What a concept!) Unfortunately, the many labels in the supermarket today are vague, skewed, and typically misleading, insinuating conditions not entirely true in order to make a profit. Here's the deal on what those labels *really* mean.

1. "USDA Organic"
"USDA Organic" is the crème de la crème of food labels, the one most regulated by the United States Department of Agriculture. It signifies how the products are raised/grown and processed. Organic products preserve natural resources and biodiversity, and are kept separate from non-organic products. The label is especially relevant from a Paleo perspective, since organic farming is intended to mimic natural, wild conditions.

Organic crops are grown in safe soil with no synthetic fertilizers, synthetic pesticides, genetically modified organisms (GMOs), or irradiation (chemically modifying the crop with radiation for preservative purposes). Consuming organic produce is important for health because it minimizes exposure to toxic pesticides, which tend to coat conventional produce (ew). You can check the non-profit *Environmental Working Group* (http://www.ewg.org/foodnews/list.php) to see which produce currently harbors the highest and lowest amounts of pesticides. As of 2015, common Paleo produce highest in pesticides were apples, strawberries, celery, spinach, blueberries, lettuce, and kale. Common Paleo produce lowest in pesticides were avocados, cabbage, asparagus, cauliflower, and sweet potatoes.

Organic meat means the animals consumed organic feed with access to the outdoors, and were given no antibiotics or growth hormones. Eating organic meat is important to minimize exposure to toxins, which accumulate in an animal's adipose tissue. Whatever the animal ingests (be it antibiotics, vitamins, Omega-3/6s, etc.) is ultimately what ends up *in you*. Because of this, fattier cuts are more "important" for the organic seal than leaner cuts. However, when it comes to meat, truly "grass-fed" (see #2) may be even more important than organic, since it signifies the type of diet consumed by the animals, which ultimately determines their nutrient levels and Omega-3/6 ratios.

While this may go without saying, a rigorous application process yields the "certified organic" seal. If you're shopping at a local farmers market, the food may indeed be "organic" without the seal. Ask away!

2. "Grass-Fed"

"Grass-fed" is a *vital* term in spirit. It means the livestock were pasture raised, which is especially important for beef, since cattle naturally consume grass. Grass-fed beef yields a much more optimal omega-3/6 ratio (1:1) than grain-fed beef (6:1). On the downside, this label does not address the use of antibiotics, pesticides, or GMOs, and the animal's diet can still be supplemented with grains if documented. This makes the less common term "grass-finished" even more important.

3. "Free-Range"

This term is positive in theory, but potentially misleading in reality. While regulated by the USDA, "free-range" simply means the animals were not caged and had access to the outdoors. Whether or not they actually ventured outside is up for debate, while the "outside" area itself could be small and netted.

4. "Cage-Free"
This term is perhaps the most misleading. It means the animals were not in literal cages and had constant access to food and water. However, they still may have been in cramped, interior spaces. In fact, the official USDA site assumes that "the flock was able to freely roam a building, room, or enclosed area" - they're not frolicking fields here, folks.

5. "Vegetarian-Fed"
This one is ridiculously misleading. I see it and laugh. It simply means exactly what it says: the animals ate vegetarian feed. This could still be GMO, or corn/soy feed, so it's rather pointless from a Paleo perspective. Grain-fed is vegetarian-fed, and we're not fans of grains around here!

6. "Natural"
This is a very vague term. By USDA standards, it only applies to meat and eggs, and simply means "minimally processed" with no artificial ingredients. Produce labeled "natural" is not regulated at all.

7. "Pasture-Raised"
This one sounds great in theory, but isn't regulated at all. Proceed with caution.

8. "No Added Hormones"
This means the animals were raised without added hormones. (Surprise, surprise.) It's really only applicable to beef or dairy products, since federal regulations have never allowed steroids or hormones in poultry, pork, or goat. Chicken with "no added hormones" is just a trick to get your money. Sneaky devils.

SAY WHAT?
If all those labels seem a little cray cray, here's a summary! "USDA Organic" is ideal for everything. For *produce,* it really is all you need. If money is an issue, refer to the "Environmental Working Group" and choose organic for the produce highest in pesticides. For *meat,* favor organic *and* preferably "grass-fed" or "grass-finished" cuts (especially for the fattier meat). Think about it this way. Plants universally "eat" sunlight, so the dangers come from whatever is put *on* them. But what an animal eats varies, and ultimately determines the nutrients, Omega-3/6 ratio, and even potential toxins in its meat. As such, the animal's diet is quite important for its nutritional value .

When all's said and done, conventional produce and meat is still better than processed foods, sugar, and grains any day! *"I can't afford organic so I'll just buy pasta"* is not a good excuse. Sorry Charlie.

Chapter Nine

Dining, Paleo Style

Dining at restaurants Paleo-style is quite feasible once you get the hang of it. Most restaurants have some sort of meat dish on the menu, as well as vegetables. You just gotta think outside the box. Paleo is also super easy because you don't have to gauge calories or scrutinize portion sizes! (*Can I get an Amen?*)

RESTAURANT PALEO PROTOCOL

1. Pick a meat dish you like.

2. Ask for sauce on the side.

3. Substitute sides for veggies.

Done.

Indeed, perhaps the most difficult thing about eating out Paleo-style isn't so much *finding* something to eat, as it is communicating with the waitstaff. You sit there *knowing* what you want to order "in theory," but are silenced by nerves, hesitancy to ask questions, and fears of being annoying. So when the time comes to order, you mumble a disheartened *"I'll take the chicken,"* and then silently pray that the sauce isn't sugar or gluten-infested.

If such is your predicament, have no fear: you simply must adopt the proper temperament. For starters, always be nice in communicating with the waitstaff. Kindness gets you far! Commence the order by sincerely saying something to the effect of, *"I'm a little crazy with my ordering, sorry!"* This acknowledges you don't *want* to be annoying, while also preparing them for the madness. (We don't want post-traumatic stress here.) After the order is complete, sincerely thank them. Make it known you appreciate their time. Consider a contrite *"Sorry about the pickiness!"* as a final touch. And don't worry about them judging you for being picky. It just doesn't matter, really.

RESTAURANT ORDERING TIPS

Utilize these tips and tricks for menu ordering, so you can publicly embrace your caveman habits. (**Note:** As I've been a waitress, I know what it's like to deal with special orders. It's doable!)

1. Substitute

Substitution is key. If you embrace substitution, you can usually Paleo-ify most dishes. Ask to substitute any "sides" (including fries!) for vegetables. I usually peruse the entire menu to see what sides *other* dishes are served with, and then request whichever veggie looks best. (Pay attention to the sides that come with the specials as well.)

If the menu says "no substitutions," ask anyway! They *usually* don't enforce that one – it's happened to me only a few times in the 5 years I've been "substituting." If they *still* insist (annoying), ask for no sides, and hope they ramp up the entrée. Or just ignore it, and don't eat the sides. No one can make you eat anything you don't want! It's your mouth and your body. Give them to someone else. Trade. Barter.

2. Simplify Veggies

You can usually get simpler versions of "complicated" vegetables. If they've got sautéed spinach for example, they can *probably* do steamed. The special has a mushroom roulade? Ask for mushrooms! The exception tends to be some mixed vegetables. If it's a cheaper restaurant, the veggies may already be pre-mixed. But always ask!

3. Sauce On The Side
Sauce and dressings are the *perfect* concoctions for hidden sugar, gluten, and processed "stuff." *Always* ask for them on the side. In fact, I do this even when I have no intention of eating the sauce. Wasteful you say? Perhaps. But I feel like it's a nod to the chef, in an *"I appreciate this sauce you have concocted"* type way. And don't stress about the inconvenience – there's often an easy "sauce on the side" button for the waitstaff to press when they input the order into the system.

4. Substitute Buns For Lettuce
I *could* put this under substitute, but it's an awesome one most people don't think about. You may feel weird, but you can pretty much always ask for sandwiches and burgers over lettuce. (A few restaurants even offer this as an option up front.) Look at sandwiches and burgers as meat & veggie plates in disguise!

5. Ask Questions
Channel grade school's *"the only stupid question is the one you didn't ask"* theme. Don't be afraid to ask questions! I always ask if the meats are prepared in anything (like marinated, breaded, or with a sauce). Ask about gluten and added sugar. Ask what type of oil they use. Ask what the "mixed vegetables" entails. (Sometimes it's only starchy vegetables, which I personally minimize.) While this may sound like a lot of questions, it's not *that* bad. Besides, you'll be tailoring the questions to your potential entrées, not running down the entire menu. If you feel awkward at any point, cite "health reasons." It's true after all!

6. Say You're Allergic
Whether you're actually "allergic" by *technical* standards may be up for debate, but it definitely eradicates feelings of being "picky," more so than the vague "health reasons" one. It also makes the waitstaff and chef more likely to honor your

wishes, since no one wants to get sued. And maybe you are actually allergic and just don't know it! I was! (*Oh hey wheat allergy!*)

7. Embrace The Unknown
Even if you don't see a specific side item on the menu, they still might have it! I've done this many a time, and have found restaurants often *do* have sides not listed. Ask away! (I don't think I've ever asked for an *entrée* not on the menu. If you do this with success, please let me know.)

8. Salad Dressings
Most salad dressings have some sort of gluten, sugar, or other nefarious ingredient in them. Favor oil and vinegar. It's the safest choice, and most restaurants have it, even if they don't list it.

9. Approach Dessert Differently
Some restaurants have fruit dessert plates, and many do cheese plates, if you're including dairy in your protocol. I typically just munch on my family's leftover meat while they eat dessert. I'm not kidding. But then again, I'm a crazy carnivore. I used to feel weird, but now it's whatever.

10. Look At The Menu Online
Most restaurants have online menus, so you can always "prepare" your choice (and salivate over it) ahead of time. I did this even before I was crazy picky. Looking at menus is fun!

11. Beware Hidden Things
This is more of a problem than you may realize. Cooking oils at restaurants can be especially problematic, while many entrées contain traces of gluten, sugar, and other things, even when you'd *least* expect it! (*Ihop* has been known to put pancake batter in their omelettes, just saying. I found that out back in my religiously ketogenic days, when I got kicked out of ketosis by an omelette. Further research revealed this nefarious tidbit of information.)

12. Consider Ordering Sides
You can always assume the "side of this, side of that" approach. In fact, ordering a ton of sides may yield more food for a cheaper price. This is especially handy for breakfast meals.

13. Don't Feel Bad
For the love of an elk, do not feel bad about being picky. Just be nice and appreciative. Consider this: if you ask a question, the server will either know or not know the answer. If they know, then what's the worry? If they don't know, they'll know next time somebody asks! You're saving them future trouble! Also, being specific up front means you will more likely be satisfied with the end result. I'm rarely ever picky when the actual food comes, because I did all the prep work! Plus, why pay good money for food which will make you sick or feel yucky afterwards?

14. Choose Your Battles
With all of this being said, sometimes it's not worth it to be *super crazy* with the substitutions and questions. If you're really only hungry for the main "Paleo" portion of your dish anyway, just go with it.

15. Live And Learn
If all of these tips make Paleo-dining look super obnoxious, have no fear! After dining out Paleo for awhile, you begin to learn how to minimize questions and annoyances while maximizing return on investment. Besides, if someone can ask how the sea bass is prepared, why can't you ask what oil they cook the meats in? (Acknowledgment of dangling preposition... and now incomplete sentence.)

RESTAURANT GENRES

Believe it or not, you can make *most* restaurants work with Paleo. Here's a guide to the genres! (All applicable restaurants, menus, etc. are current as of the publication date.)

EASIER RESTAURANTS

1. Self-Proclaimed "Healthy" Restaurants
This may go without saying, but any restaurant which prides itself on organic, "fresh," sustainable, or local-farming options is usually a winner. The food choices are typically more Paleo-friendly, with the staff "understanding" of substitutions. The caveat is *Vegan/Vegetarian* restaurants, as discussed in a bit.

2. Steakhouses
These are my go-to restaurants for Paleo. Show me a steakhouse that doesn't have meat and veggies? Enough said.

3. Seafood Restaurants
Like steakhouses, seafood places also tend to be great, featuring fish and vegetables.

4. Italian, French, Mediterranean
People may say these are difficult, but in my experience they usually have meat entrées, as well as vegetable options.

5. BBQ
These are *usually* good, but make sure to inquire about the "rubs" used on the meats (sneaky gluten and sugar!) It can be surprisingly difficult to get meat at BBQ places without sugar or gluten.

MORE DIFFICULT RESTAURANTS

1. Korean BBQ
You'd *think* Korean BBQ would be easy, but I *always* get sick after it. Cross contamination seems to be a thing. Make sure to avoid marinated meats, and try to cook on your own "section" of the grill, no matter how weird it feels. The type of Korean BBQ where you cook in water (rather than on a grill) tends to be a safer choice.

2. Mexican
Staple Mexican dishes feature tortillas and sauces, while go-to sides are rice and beans, none of which are Paleo-friendly. Consider salads, fajitas without the beans, or carnitas (although good luck with avoiding gluten exposure). Some Mexican chains feature gluten-free menus, à la *Blue Mesa Grill, Moe's Southwest Grill, On The Border,* and *Rubio's.*

3. Japanese
Like Mexican, Japanese also features many hard to avoid sauces. It *can* be ok with meat and vegetables, especially at the cook-in-front-of-you types, but gluten exposure is still a problem.

4. Chinese
Chinese can be really tough. Most dishes feature unavoidably combined food items in sauces. Trying to figure out what the menu actually means, coupled with the language barrier, doesn't help either. If you *have* to do Chinese, consider a chain with a gluten-free menu, à la *Pei Wei* or *P.F. Chang's.*

5. German
I realize most people don't typically dine German-style, but since I'm German, I thought I'd include it for grins. German is pretty difficult, featuring sausages with questionable additives and breaded meats. This section is massively unhelpful I guess.

6. Tapas
Tapas restaurants can be misleadingly difficult. They typically prepare the individual tapas *very* delicately with sauces, seasonings, and specific ingredients, so substituting just seems weird for such a small portion. Plus, as you're often sharing said food with other people, you may feel more self-conscious about making your health concerns known.

7. Vegan, Vegetarian
While at first you may think #*healthy!*, vegan and vegetarian places can actually be quite tricky. While this goes without saying, there are no meat dishes to form the bulk of your meal. Many dishes also rely on problematic components like

grains, legumes, and tofu. While you can likely find something to eat, you may walk away less than satisfied.

$$$

In general, fancier and more expensive restaurants tend to be more accommodating to special requests, while also using less additives and processed ingredients. On the flip side, fixed price menus at such places are typically not kind to substitutions, while also "forcing" you to get a dessert. The uber expensive ones can also be annoying when the celebrity chef has concocted the "perfect" entrée which would *never* entertain substitutions.

CHAINS

Most sit-down chains in America (think *Chili's*, *Red Lobster*, and *TGI Fridays*) regulate their menus to minimize the hassle of dealing with picky eaters all over the country, making them surprisingly Paleo-friendly. Since they have a built-in audience and are not trying to "prove a point" food wise with the vigor of an independent restaurant, chains are also pretty understanding of substitutions. Some feature easy "mix-and-match" type menus with the whole meat and veggie thing, à la *Outback Steakhouse*. My favorite chains for Paleo concoctions are *Cheesecake Factory*, *Seasons 52*, and *Bonefish*.

Many chains even feature *gluten-free menus!* These are fantastic, although they *do* make you realize just how many things *aren't* gluten-free. (*You mean this chicken isn't gluten-free? Oh.*) Restaurants with gluten-free menus include *Applebee's*, *BJ's*, *Bob Evans*, *Buffalo Wild Wings*, *Carrabba's*, *Chili's*, *Denny's*, *Domino's*, *Fleming's*, *Logan's Roadhouse*, *LongHorn*, *Olive Garden*, *On The Border*, *Outback Steakhouse*, *Pei Wei*, *Perkins*, *P.F. Chang's*, *Red Lobster*, *Red Robin*, *Roy's Hawaiian Fusion*, *Ruby Tuesday*, *Togo's*, and *Yard House*, along with many others. As always, never be afraid to ask!

FAST FOOD

While I shudder stepping foot in them, Paleo can still be done fast food-style, and the fact that you can typically look up the "nutrition" facts for carb and sodium content is a nice touch. When "dining" fast food-style, favor salads. This is super easy at places like *Subway*, but you can still go this route at *McDonalds*. "Bowls" at places like *Chipotle* or *Freebirds* are also a win! Be wary of breading. (*Chick-fil-A's* chicken nuggets, while delicious, are a no-go. Try their salad with grilled chicken instead.)

Some fast food places also have *secret menus* which are way more Paleo friendly! *Panera Bread*, for example, has a "Power Menu" featuring high protein and salad options, like a "Power Breakfast Bowl" with egg, steak, avocado, and tomato, and a "Power Steak Lettuce Wrap" with steak, lettuce, and veggie garnishes! (I find it ironic that a chain with the word "bread" in the title, chooses the word "power" for menu items that include... no bread.) *In-N-Out's* "Not-So-Secret-Menu" lets you order burgers "Protein Style" (the bun is switched for lettuce), "Double Meat" (double the meat, no cheese), or "3x3s"/"4x4s" (which increases the number of burger patties by that number). Even *Taco Bell* recently jumped on the Paleo bandwagon with their "Cantina Power Menu," featuring protein-heavy items with double the meat, but still under 500 calories. (That's just how they're pitching it – we Paleo people laugh in the face of calories!)

DISNEY DINING

Because I'm obsessed with Disney, it gets its own section! You can always order off the kid's menu, which typically features very simple concoctions. And customizing meals can save you money: asking for no sides at counter service places makes the meal cheaper! Perhaps most importantly, never buy bottled water in the parks: they'll give you free cups of water at all counter service places! Actually, this really has nothing to do with Paleo, I just love Disney.

CHAPTER TEN

PALEO ADHERENCE TIPS

Changing habits is hard. *Especially* when those habits involve food. Not to mention that the super palatable, refined, processed foods we eat today function psychology like an addiction, which doesn't help matters. But while going Paleo may be an uphill journey, it *will* be worth it! I wouldn't be so enthusiastic about Paleo if it hadn't literally changed my life. I didn't make a website or write a book or engage in epic research and diet discussions when I tried calorie counting or the "cookie diet" or vegetarianism. Although the transition to Paleo may seem difficult at first, the "other side" is so beautiful when you get there! Once you have practiced Paleo for a bit and experienced the benefits, you will begin to realize how crappy sugar and processed foods make you feel, while whole foods fill you with health and vitality! Be passionate, reflective, and real. Take it one step at a time! Try these tips to help you adhere to the Paleo lifestyle!

1. Mindset
Proper mindset is key. Do Paleo for health, not weight loss. The weight loss will come, trust me, but if you're doing Paleo

for weight loss *only*, you may feel more "restricted," since we're conditioned to believe weight loss is a torturous path. (Although it doesn't have to be, as I'm attempting to show you.) Viewing Paleo as a health choice renders it more "positive" in your mind. Here's a fun mind trick: Say "I don't" instead of "I can't." For example, replace *"I can't eat sugar"* with *"I don't eat sugar."* Studies show this simple change in terminology actually *increases* willpower by making the decision a choice rather than a restriction. Pretty cool.

2. Remove Temptation
Clear your cabinets of processed foods. It doesn't matter how strong your willpower may be: if it's there, *you will want it*. (Speaking from experience here.) If you simply *can't* throw something away, put it somewhere hard to reach, like a shelf requiring a step ladder, or buried behind boxes in a cabinet. After being Paleo for awhile, you'll likely find newfound inspiration to toss the toxic goods.

3. Be Simple
Err on the side of simplicity. As your tastebuds change from going Paleo, you'll find you don't need an abundance of salt, sugar, and flavorings for food to taste good. Embrace this "simple" change. Combining lots of ingredients to make things super palatable can actually interfere with appetite regulation. If you favor a more basic and "clean" approach to meals, you may just find yourself more satisfied in the end. A basic Paleo meal, for example, can consist of some meat, coconut oil, and veggies! Before Paleo, I couldn't imagine eating naked meats not slathered in sauces. I now actually prefer meats completely au naturel, with no sauces or seasonings added! That being said, adding some simple spices, like turmeric or ginger, can make meals not only super delicious, but even more healthy to boot!

4. Avoid Mimicking Old Habits
Don't fall into the trap of substituting to mimic old food choices. When you keep tempting treats in your life like sugar substitutes and Paleo-ified baking recipes, you may continue to crave the foods they are replacing. Consider being bold and eradicating all hints of your former cravings and

temptations. Save the Paleo-friendly dessert substitutions (which often taste *fabulous* by the way) for special occasions. I personally found that the stricter I became, the easier it was to adhere. Look for *new food possibilities*, not new versions of old ones.

5. *Remember that nothing tastes as good as healthy feels!*

6. Plan Ahead
Consider planning your meals ahead of time. Rather than waiting till you get to the kitchen when you're hungry, decide beforehand what you'll be eating the next few meals. Same with the grocery shopping. This relates to a concept known as "ego depletion" or "decision fatigue," in which the more choices you make, the less "willpower" you have. If you're making less actual choices when it comes time to shop and eat, you'll be more likely to stick with your goals.

7. Embrace Leftovers
Consider making more than needed for dinner, and then eating leftovers for lunch, or even breakfast! The less time spent mulling over making food, the easier it is to just eat and go on with your life!

8. Companionship
Try out Paleo with a friend! If you can find someone to embark on the Paleo adventure with you, it'll be *so* much easier, motivational, and amazing! Plus you won't feel weird making special orders when dining out. Things are less embarrassing with friends!

9. Bring Your Own Food
If you work in an office setting, consider bringing your lunch (at least in the beginning), or trying some intermittent fasting, which will be discussed thoroughly in Part 2! (See Chapter 12: *What Is Intermittent Fasting* if you just can't wait!) If you bring your own lunch, you won't be as tempted by cafeteria food. For parties, bring a "party favor" of Paleo-friendly food. Of course, once you get used to Paleo, you'll have much more self control and be able to laugh in the face of any food temptations present.

10. Distractions
Use distractions to your advantage. If you find yourself craving a candy bar or something else non-Paleo, use it as an excuse to do something distracting which you love. Your brain is probably just craving some dopamine, so get it some other way! Watch that Netflix! Go for a walk. Text your crush. Dance around your room to some super motivating song. (Confession: I do that last one a lot.)

11. Find A Paleo Snack
Find a Paleo-friendly snack you love, so you'll always have something to munch on! Veggies like cucumbers, celery, and kale chips are great! Nuts are nice too. (Just don't, as Robb Wolf often points out, consume a Costco-sized tub of almonds in one sitting.)

12. Prevent Cravings
Try to minimize factors which cause cravings. Stress and lack of sleep, while hard to avoid at times, notably encourage mindless eating signals. Try to get your sleep (*I know, I know*) and find ways to manage stress, be it through yoga, meditation, prayer, exercise, talking to family, or simply laughing with friends.

13. Avoid The Scale
For the love of a bison, please do not use the scale. If you must, step on it once a week or so. You shouldn't be judging progress by a scale number, especially since it says *nothing* of body composition and can be quite misleading in regards to fat and muscle. A person's scale weight is also easily swayed by fluctuating water levels and hormones, especially for females. Instead of a certain scale number, judge by how your clothes fit, how you look in the mirror, and how you feel. (Which will be increasingly awesome!)

14. Record Your Journey
Consider taking "before and after" pictures for motivation! Journal along the way! Blog! Write a book! Keeping a tangible record of your journey can remind you of your progress for those times when motivation wanes.

15. *Reflect on how awesome it is to not count calories!*

16. Research
If you're the information-lover type, research and read all you can about the science of Paleo. You'll understand *why* Paleo is so amazing for health, making you that much more excited and committed. You'll also pick up many tips along the way and feel less alone in choosing a healthy lifestyle, which can definitely happen whenever you go against the norm.

17. Deal With Peer Pressure
If you're feeling pressured by others to break your diet, consider why. It may be for their *own* satisfaction, not yours. (*"Oh you have to try this cake"* translates to *"You have to try this cake so I won't feel bad about eating it."*) People like to make dieters feel bad by "making food such a big deal," when really *they're* the ones making a big deal of the situation. Perhaps they don't want to feel guilty about their own choices, or feel uncomfortable with your "drastic" change. Just remember *you* are in control of what you eat. And you can do it! There are a lot of worse struggles out there.

18. Salivate
Chances are, if you've "dieted" in the past, you're probably accustomed to lackluster fat-free frankenfoods which never satisfy. With Paleo, you can eat a steak, and enjoy it! Relish the moment!

19. Imagine
When you *really* want to eat that cookie, think ahead to your happy, healthy self. The one who didn't give in. Find a go-to happy place in your mind for when you're struggling. Studies have shown that imagination can promote perceived plausibility of an event by changing judgements and behavior. This means if you imagine your "happy, healthy self," you're more likely to believe you can *become* that happy, healthy self, which massively aids diet adherence. A 2011 study found that imagination actually influences perception of the real world. In other words, consciously imaging things

influences how you *literally* see them. I have this weird imagination game where I imagine myself on an amazing date with someone I have a major crush on, and everybody looks beautiful, and I'm happy and healthy. It nips cravings in the bud for me.

20. Never Beat Yourself Up!

Whatever you do, do not beat yourself up about anything! You are a beautiful human being, and scolding yourself for a diet slip is just silly. It won't kill you, and you can still make progress! See it as a learning experience. *("Well, we won't be doing that again!")* Whenever I slip up, instead of being like, "*You've already messed up, so might as well eat all the sugar!*" I like to think, "*It can only go up from here!*"

CHAPTER ELEVEN

PALEO Q&A

Got Paleo questions? Here's some answers! For unaddressed thoughts, feel free to contact me via *WhatWhenWine.com*.

PALEO PROTOCOL QUESTIONS

What Should My Macronutrient Ratio Be On A Paleo Diet?
This is a common question on the Paleo diet. How much protein, carbs, and fat should you consume? High carb or low carb? High fat or low fat? Paleo tends to provide adequate levels of the various macronutrients without much "thought" required. As Robb Wolf says, Paleo is "macronutrient agnostic." Once you leave behind the confusing signals of processed food and refined sugar, and balance your blood sugar levels, you will likely find your body naturally tells you what to eat. Cravings become signs of actual nutritional needs, rather than junk food-driven assaults from your brain's reward center demanding another hit of dopamine. (I find that I now specifically

crave protein, fat, or carbs based on the current nutritional need of my body.)

If you would like to measure macronutrient intake, focus on adequate protein as a foundation: around 1 gram of protein per pound of lean body mass per day. Fill out the rest of your daily food intake with fats and carbs from there, based on your preference. Eat to satiety.

I personally choose a higher fat, lower carb approach, favoring green vegetables and oils, rather than fruit and starchy Paleo-friendly carbs like sweet potatoes and squash. I love the consistent energy levels that come from functioning almost solely from fats, and it pairs especially well with my fasting habits. That being said, you can definitely do a higher carb version of Paleo with starchy veggies. (And indeed, this will still likely be lower in carbs than the typical Standard American Diet.) The increased insulin sensitivity from Paleo makes the body more adept at utilizing carbs to replenish muscle glycogen and fulfill nutritional needs, rather than merely storing them as fat. Feel it out for yourself. Focus on adequate protein, and then see if you function better on more fat, or more carbs.

Can I Have Cheat Meals?

Although I have definitely indulged in my fair share of them, I strongly advise against cheat meals, at least as a "written" part of your protocol. Cheating tends to keep cravings present, making the transition to Paleo uncomfortable, and postponing your ultimate freedom from grain and sugar addiction. Furthermore, an introduction period (preferably 30 days) is vital to eliminate all potentially problematic and inflammatory aspects of your diet. Seemingly minor exposures to problematic foods can yield substantial allergic and immune responses, so cheating here and there while transitioning can sustain inflammation.

But if you do indeed cheat, don't beat yourself up! You're only human! Don't fall into the *"I just had a cookie so I might as well eat* EVERYTHING *I can since I already messed up"* mindset. You'll feel better the day after a minor slip than a major one. If you broke your arm, would you say, *"Well, might as well break every other limb since I'm already broken"*? Doubt it.

Do I Need To Take Supplements?

In a perfect world, a whole foods diet would provide all the nutrients we need. However, much has gone askew in our modern, processed world, so this isn't necessarily the case. Toxins, skewed Omega-3/6 ratios, the chronic stress of modern life, the influx of antibiotic use, and high grain intakes, have all lead to damaged guts less adept at nutrient assimilation. Supplements can fill in gaps and deficiencies, enhance performance, and just increase vitality in general.

Of course there are many supplements out there (coming from a supplement freak here), so what's most important? While individual needs vary, here are my three favorites if I had to pick:

> 1. *Omega-3* supplementation via fish or flaxseed oil to help balance today's inflammatory Omega-3/6 ratio.
>
> 2. A *probiotic* to restore and maintain healthy gut flora damaged from antibiotics and food choices.
>
> 3. If you're not getting sunshine (at least 10 minutes or so a day), definitely consider some *vitamin D!* In fact, take it even if you are a sun god or goddess!

Beyond these three, feel free to research and try different supplements to fit your individual needs!

PALEO FOOD QUESTIONS

How Much Fruit Can I Eat On A Paleo Diet?

The amount of fruit to consume on a Paleo diet sparks constant debate. To be completely clear, fruit IS Paleo. Fruit is a whole food, and definitely the route to take for those moments you're hankering for something sweet. That being said, present day fruit has been selectively bred to be quite sweet, often at the expense of nutrients. (The banana, for example, is a selectively-bred seedless, sterile fruit which was originally inedible due to its seeds.) As for the sweetness, fruit is notably high in fructose, which is processed primarily by the liver and encourages fat storage, fails to instigate satiety signals, and contributes to non-alcoholic fatty liver disease. (It is unreliable for refilling muscle glycogen specifically, if such is your intention. Starchy vegetables are a better route for that.) Non-organic fruit is also often coated in "nontoxic" toxic pesticides, as well as wax to retain moisture, protect it from bruising, and make it look pretty.

The amount of fruit you consume will likely depend on whether you choose a higher or lower carb Paleo approach. I've been low carb for so long, that I'm much more comfortable without fruit, which tends to spike my blood sugar, especially if consumed when fasted. The most Paleo-friendly fruits are low in sugar but high in nutrients and antioxidants. This includes berries (like raspberries, cranberries, blueberries, and blackberries), apples, pears, and grapefruit. Avoid high glycemic index fruits such as melons and bananas, and especially refined versions of fruits such as dried fruit or fruit juices, which often feature higher glycemic indexes and less nutrition.

What's The Deal On Dairy?

Dairy makes the "maybe" list, and is widely debated in the Paleo world. Dairy is not "Paleo" in the sense that Paleolithic people did not consume it (besides breast milk I guess). Beyond that, many people react negatively to dairy. Those who are lactose-intolerant lack the enzyme needed to break down the lactose (sugar) in milk, which can lead to digestive issues such as gas and bloating. Others are allergic to the casein (protein) in milk, which can be a potent histamine releaser. Still others are allergic to whey (the liquid part of milk). Cheese can also be *extremely addicting* on a neurological level. It contains casomorphin peptides (protein fragments coming from casein) which have an opioid-like effect on the brain. (When I found that out, I was just like, *"That makes so much sense."*) Milk is also highly insulinogenic, promoting insulin release and inflammation. Lastly, dairy increases mucous production and may encourage acne.

I recommend excluding dairy completely for the first 30 days, and then reintroducing it if desired to see how you react. While I'm not specifically allergic to dairy, I still feel better consuming less of it. It was one of the last things to go (cream in my coffee and cheese), but now that I've cut it out, I don't struggle with its negative effects of excess mucous production and breakouts. That being said, I can definitely handle a little dairy here or there, and use cheese as a splurge "dessert" on occasion. If you do choose to eat dairy, favor organic, raw, and fermented varieties. Full fat yogurt with live cultures is notably good for repopulating gut flora.

What Are Nightshades?

Nightshades are a group of plants containing naturally occurring "soapy" alkaloids called *saponins*, which serve as protective mechanisms against fungi. (They get their name from the "soapwort" plant used to make soap.) Common nightshades include sweet and hot peppers, tomatoes, potatoes, and eggplant. Saponins may irritate the respiratory and digestive tract, inhibit digestive enzymes and nutrient uptake, encourage leaky gut, and yield an immune response and inflammation. As not everyone reacts negatively to nightshades, feel free to reintroduce them individually after 30 days of strict Paleo, and see how you react. Cooking nightshades can help neutralize negative effects.

What Are Cruciferous Vegetables?

Cruciferous vegetables are a group of veggies containing protective chemicals called *glucosinolates* which can affect the thyroid. Common cruciferous vegetables include broccoli, Brussels sprouts, cabbage, and Bok Choy. Glucosinolates act as goitrogens. They can inhibit direct thyroid processes and block iodine absorption necessary for proper thyroid function. (The thyroid gland produces thyroxine (T-4) and triiodothyronine (T-3) hormones which affect metabolism and energy production, protein synthesis, body temperature, and heart rate.) Anti-thyroid compounds may also encourage goiter, an enlarged state of the thyroid, while iodine deficiencies may slow sexual and mental maturation. An estimate of more than one billion people are at risk of thyroid disfunction. In fact, research suggests we even have a taste receptor (hTAS2R38) that detects glucosinolates in food. If you're particularly sensitive to glucosinolates, foods containing them may literally taste more bitter to you than to someone not as sensitive. Although cruciferous vegetables are quite nutritious, you may not want to binge on them per se, especially if you react negatively. Cooking cruciferous vegetables can help neutralize negative effects.

Can I Use "Natural" Sugars Like Honey Or Agave Syrup?

Agave syrup is bad news. It can be up to 90% fructose, which encourages fat storage, non-alcoholic fatty liver disease, and a multitude of other nasty things. (See Chapter 3: *Sweet Problems* for more on the matter.) As for honey, I really don't recommend using any sort of sugar to sweeten food, even if it is "natural." Sugar in general is pretty nasty stuff, and things like honey just stir the fire. Nutrient wise, there's nothing special in honey that you can't get from whole foods. If you must sweeten something, I recommend stevia.

What About Artificial Sweeteners?

The various artificial sweeteners on the market (like aspartame, saccharin, and sucralose) interact differently within the body, and vary in their effects. While most are low on the glycemic index and do not substantially raise blood sugar, they still are processed, chemical creations not at all "Paleo" in spirit. While the majority of studies do not link them to negative effects (which surprised me), the jury is still out. They also may negatively affect a person's gut flora. Ultimately, using sweeteners tends to mimic nefarious food habits (like the desire for sweet things and dessert), and can keep cravings present. If you must use artificial sweeteners, err on the side of more "natural" ones, and avoid added fillers. I recommend stevia (*SweetLeaf* is a good brand, available in both powder and liquid form), followed by sugar alcohols such as xylitol or erythritol. Potential problems with these, however, include an allergy to stevia (particularly if you are allergic to the ragweed family), and a laxative effect from sugar alcohols if over-consumed.

What About Omega-3/Omega-6 Ratios?

The Polyunsaturated Omega-3 and Omega-6 fats (PUFAs) are the two essential fatty acids (EFAs) necessary for health which the body cannot produce on its own, and therefore must be obtained from diet. Omega-3s contain *alpha-linolenic acid* (ALA) and are found primarily in fish like salmon, herring, and tuna, with vegetable sources including walnut and flaxseed oil. As for other meats, beef is higher in Omega-3s than poultry. Omega-6 fatty acids contain *linoleic acid* (LA) and are found primarily in seed and vegetable oils like corn, soybean, and safflower oil. Omega-6 fats are notably concentrated in processed foods.

While both essential, Omega-6s are pro-inflammatory, while Omega-3s are anti-inflammatory. Historically, hunter-gatherers consumed these fats in a balanced 1:1 ratio, negating detrimental effects. Today's modern diet rampant in grain, wheat, and seed oils, however, has encouraged diets high in inflammatory Omega-6s and low in anti-inflammatory Omega-3s. In fact, the typical Omega-6:3 ratio of today's Western diet may be as high as 16:1! Even natural sources of Omega-3s such as meat have become skewed towards the Omega-6 side, thanks to grain-based diets fed to the animals. This high Omega-6 diet generates inflammation in the body. The increased levels of Omega-6s have been linked to the pathogenesis of many cardiovascular, inflammatory, and autoimmune diseases, as well as cancer. On the flip side, increasing Omega-3s yields a protective effect against such diseases.

To help balance your Omega-3:6 ratio, minimize grains and vegetable/seed oils, and favor fatty fish. You can also take fish oil supplements.

What About Fiber?

Fiber refers to indigestible carbohydrates found in the cell walls of plants. Although fiber adds no real caloric or nutritional value to food, it serves as a bulking agent (good for satiety), regulates digestion, and feeds gut flora. There are two types of fiber: *soluble fiber*, which dissolves in water and bulks up in your system, and *insoluble fiber*, which does not dissolve in water, and basically passes through you unchanged. Don't worry about getting enough fiber without grains. Calorie for calorie, the amount of fiber in green vegetables outweighs that of grains. On a 100 calorie basis, bread contains around 1.5-3 grams of fiber, while green vegetables such as broccoli and spinach contain 7-10 grams. Paleo foods high in fiber include green vegetables, squash, sweet potatoes, avocados, and fruits such as apples and berries. And all that being said, fiber's benefits may be slightly overhyped. See Chapter 2: *Grainy Problems* for more on that!

What About Calcium?

Adequate calcium intake builds strong bones and teeth, while supporting nervous system, heart, and muscular health. Calcium needs to be properly balanced with magnesium (1:1) and vitamin D to ensure proper absorption. Paleo foods rich in calcium include nuts, vegetables, and oily fish; magnesium is found in many nuts and vegetables; and vitamin D comes from sunshine and oily fish. Eating a mixed Paleo diet thus encourages an ideal calcium/magnesium/vitamin D ratio for proper calcium absorption!

A Paleo diet is also one step ahead with calcium, as it encourages calcium absorption. Anti-nutrients in a typical diet (such as phytates in grains and legumes), too much salt, or even too much fiber, can actually encourage calcium excretion. And while dairy provides an abundance of calcium, too much calcium at one time from dairy may actually reduce its absorption by up to 75%.

PALEO DRINK QUESTIONS

How Much Water Should I Be Drinking?

Before I was Paleo, I often wondered if I was drinking "enough" water. Now, the question seems almost odd to me. When you're eating hydrating whole fruits and vegetables, while not consuming processed foods high in sodium, the whole water thing becomes second nature! Drink so you don't feel thirsty. And if you're thirsty, drink water! The body is pretty good at relaying thirst signals, which don't get screwed up like food signals. Don't fear the water, but don't stress about filling some "magical water quota" either. Contrary to popular belief, thirst does not mean you're already dehydrated.

Note: You may need more water if you're doing a super low carb version of Paleo. Glucose is stored with water as glycogen, while fat is "hydrophobic." Low carb diets thus require more supplementation with water. This is also why you can lose or gain a good amount of "weight" unnaturally fast when shifting carb intakes. The initial weight change is mostly water.

Can I Have Tea Or Coffee?

Surely! Tea boasts many antioxidant, anti-aging, and other health benefits. Besides the cognitive benefits from caffeine, green tea in particular contains a catechin called EGCG (epigallocatechin gallate), a potent antioxidant, with strong anti-cancer properties, and which may inhibit fat gain and reduce fatigue. Green tea also promotes cardiac health, reduces oxidative stress, and helps regulate cholesterol.

Coffee, the world's second beverage behind water, yields many health benefits, but also problematic side effects. Its active compounds include caffeine and chlorogenic acid. Coffee consumption can help reduce oxidative stress, support brain functioning, and may be preventative against diabetes, cancers, Parkinson's disease, and Alzheimer's. On the other hand, too much coffee consumption may raise cholesterol, instigate cardiovascular problems, and encourage jitters and insomnia. Coffee's high caffeine content also easily promotes tolerance (so you require more and more to reach the same "level" of stimulation), as well as withdrawal symptoms when cut out.

The benefits of tea and coffee seem to outweigh the side effects, if consumed in moderation. Just make sure you don't load them with with cream (if you're avoiding dairy), sugar, or artificial sweeteners. If you must sweeten them, try more Paleo-friendly sweeteners such as stevia.

What Is Bulletproof Coffee?

A lot of people in the Paleo community consume bulletproof coffee: coffee with a tablespoon or so of added MCT oil or ghee/butter popularized by Dave Asprey. Many find bulletproof coffee leads to sustained energy levels throughout the day, with less jitters and "crashing." I used to partake when I drank more coffee, and rather fancied it. The butter thing sounds weird, but it actually makes the coffee quite creamy and tasty. Bulletproof coffee is also highly satiating.

What About Juice Cleanses?

I'm on the fence about juice cleanses. On the one hand, if you've been following a typical Standard American Diet, and then commence a juice cleanse, you'll likely see benefits. The nature of the cleanse eliminates a vast amount of problematic substances ingested prior to that point. The inevitable calorie restriction can also be a good thing. If you're already Paleo however, it's more of a grey area. With juice cleanses, you'll be running almost entirely on sugar, even if you're only drinking "green juices." Although the inevitable calorie deficit may negate any deleterious effects (as the sugar is burned more immediately, leaving less room for damage), I still prefer complete fasting à la intermittent fasting, as discussed in Part II!

Personally, I think juice cleanses might be good if you're the extremist type (like me) who needs something "drastic" to change your mindset, or if you need some sort of "cleanse" to transition into a healthier lifestyle. I doubt juice cleanses will harm you, and they might even help you - I just believe their benefits may be attributed to the wrong reasons.

What About Alcohol?

In the strict Paleo world, alcohol is a no-go; however, many Paleo people leave wiggle room for this fourth macronutrient. (I've even heard the argument that Paleolithic man and animals would consume alcohol via fermented fruit.) Studies consistently link moderate alcohol consumption to a myriad of health benefits, specifically heart health and longevity. I vote consume alcohol in moderation if you so desire. (Which you probably guessed, given the title of this book.)

Red wine in particular vastly enhances health, thanks to its many polyphenols, such as the heralded resveratrol. If you prefer something stronger, choose clear liquors (like gin, vodka, or tequila) sipped straight, or paired with non-offensive mixers like club soda and lime. The "Norcal Margarita" is a common drink in Paleoland, consisting of tequila, lime juice/pulp, and club soda to taste.

PRACTICAL PALEO QUESTIONS

How Long Will It Take To Start Seeing Benefits From Paleo?

It's hard for me to give a personal testimonial on this issue. I had cleaned up my diet substantially via low carb before starting Paleo, so full blown Paleo was like the icing on the cake. If you're already low carb, or sugar/gluten-free, the transition may be a breeze! My sister, for example, originally went gluten-free before trying Paleo. It took her a few months to adjust to gluten-free, but then just a few days for Paleo. When my mom tried Paleo (so exciting!), she experienced benefits within a couple of days! As my friend Kara says,

> That's a hard question to answer. In some ways the answer is about 5 days, once the bloating from my crap diet went away, and I kind of magically got a bit leaner. In some ways the answer is it took me closer to a year to really embrace the lifestyle and stop cheating so much. And in some ways the answer is that sometimes it's still hard and can backfire, especially if I'm training and go too low carb accidentally.

From the many Paleo testimonials I've read, and from friends' experiences, expect to see changes in a few days at the earliest, a few weeks at the latest! If you're starting cold turkey from a Standard American Diet, you'll probably get your first boost of motivation in a few days, when, as Kara noted, the bloating from a processed diet subsides, and you get "magically" leaner all of a sudden. A good moment indeed!

I Just Started Paleo And Feel Like Crap. Why?

If you've never been low carb before, or aren't very accustomed to using fats as fuel, you may initially experience "low carb flu" when first starting Paleo. These are withdrawal-like symptoms of fatigue as your body protests giving up sugar as fuel, like a crying baby. Don't worry - they WILL go away! If you stick it out, your body will upregulate metabolic pathways for using dietary and body fat as energy, and you'll eventually experience an amazing, sustained energy free from blood sugar crashes and constant hunger. Any perceived struggle is completely worth it! Thankfully, not everyone experiences withdrawal symptoms: I didn't when I first went low carb.

How Do I Shop Paleo?

When shopping Paleo-style, you'll mostly walk around the outer perimeter of the store, in the produce and meat departments. Venture into the aisles for healthy oils, or a nice bottle of red wine. Avoid buying things with added ingredients. Think of yourself as a modern day hunter-gatherer, seeking out fresh food! Of course you can also stock up on frozen vegetables, and buy meat in bulk. Consider trying out local farmers markets! See Chapter 8: *Shopping, Paleo Style* for more tips!

How Will I Have Time For Cooking Paleo?

Just because you won't be eating many instant microwave meals or packaged foods when doing Paleo, doesn't mean it has to be time consuming! You simply must re-evaluate the situation and embrace a bit of pre-planning. Many fruits, vegetables, and oils are ready-to-eat in their present state. As for meats, you can always cook a large amount at once and refrigerate or freeze leftovers for later. Places like *Trader Joe's* have many easy meal options, especially frozen ones.

Consider new methods of cooking. I love using a steamer: not only is it a super healthy way to cook, but it's insanely easy as well! Just throw in meat and vegetables, and let it handle the cooking! Crockpots are also a great way to throw in a bunch of ingredients in the morning, and come home to a yummy dinner! Plus if you cook a whole chicken yourself, you can use the bones for bone broth! The George Foreman grill is also a lifesaver.

And of course, if you try out intermittent fasting (the next section!), then you'll probably *gain* time when all's said and done!

Isn't Paleo Expensive?

Just because you can't live off ramen noodles and cereal while doing Paleo, doesn't mean Paleo has to be incredibly expensive. First of all, you won't be stocking up on a myriad of snacks, which saves money. You won't be buying overpriced packets of candy here and there, which sneakily add up. You don't have to worry about filling the cart to the brim with a never-ending supply of tempting things you'll "probably" eat at some point, but which ultimately end up going bad. Paleo forces you to shop wisely. Since it's mostly meat and produce, it requires you to shop on a more immediate basis. You'll likely use everything you buy without much waste, if any. Stock up on frozen veggies, and buy meat in bulk. Your fridge and freezer are your friends! See Chapter 8: *Shopping, Paleo Style* for more tips.

How Will I Eat At Restaurants?
This daunting question turns out to be fairly easy. Dining out Paleo-style really isn't difficult. Most restaurants have meat and vegetables somewhere on the menu, and you can usually substitute to "Paleo-ify" a dish. (Don't feel bad about special orders: you're the customer!) In fact, eating out Paleo-style is easier than most "diets," because you don't have to gauge calories or scrutinize portion sizes! Check out Chapter 9: *Dining, Paleo Style* for more tips!

How Will I Live Without Sugar, Cake, and Bread?
When I say my favorite meal used to be pasta, Coca-Cola, and cake… I mean my favorite meal used to be pasta, Coca-Cola, and cake. I could *never* imagine a world without carbs and sweets. The idea of *not* choosing a pasta dish, or saying *no* to dessert was laughable. Preposterous. Not gonna happen. I though people who engaged in such actions were "born that way" as health freaks. Yet today I do it with ease!

It's all about reprograming your body and brain. Grains and sugars (carbohydrates) are hard to resist because our body likes being lazy and utilizing glucose for fuel. Once it adjusts to running on fatty acids, carb cravings diminish. Furthermore, refined and processed foods are hard to give up because they trigger dopamine reward pathways in our brain - the same ones affected by alcohol and drugs.

If you abstain long enough and eat healthy, nutritious, whole foods, you *can* change your body and mind! You really *will* be able to pass on grains and sugar without experiencing an insatiable longing. Five years ago, I would have laughed at such claims, but I now experience them first hand. I'm even at the point where I can aesthetically and "vicariously" appreciate such foods through other people, without feeling deprived, lacking, or wanting. Since my body is accustomed to running on fats, and I've reprogrammed my brain's food reward system, I no longer crave them. Honestly. It happens!

Part Two
When?

CHAPTER TWELVE

WHAT IS INTERMITTENT FASTING

Intermittent fasting is a pattern of eating in which you restrict the hours you eat, rather than the quantity of food you eat. It is not so much a diet, as a diet pattern. Individual "eating windows" and timing of fasting vary. Some people implement it daily, while others use it more occasionally. I've been intermittent fasting since 2011, and personally practice it by eating all of my daily nutrition at night in a flexible dinner window. You can experiment with different IF patterns to find what works best for you! (See Chapter 13: *How To Do Intermittent Fasting* for more.)

You may be thinking:

> *"Skipping meals is bad for me. My metabolism will slow down. I will be miserable and hungry. I will lose muscle. When I begin eating again, I will store it all as fat."*

Such are the typical thoughts regarding any sort of fasting.

Contrary to popular belief, your metabolism will NOT shut down if you don't eat every 3 hours. You will not starve. (You fast every night when sleeping, and that seems to work ok.) Fasting is actually incredibly beneficial to your body. It is a hormetic stress, or "good stress," like exercise. Fasting promotes longevity, encourages insulin sensitivity, stimulates Human Growth Hormone (HGH) release and autophagy, as well as a myriad of other things. Details on all that to come.

To address one of the biggies, fasting does NOT make you tired or lethargic. With the central nervous system and body functions fueled by a steady stream of fatty acids and ketones (which we shall discuss), the fasted state is actually quite alert and energized. Rather than constantly oscillating between the fasted and fed states (and suffering blood sugar swings and mood changes), energy levels remain stable. In the fasted state, the body utilizes primarily stored fat, with all energy dedicated to activity and the immune system, rather than digestion and nutrient processing. (Eating demands a great deal of energy, which is why you may get tired after a big meal.)

I adore intermittent fasting because it gives me more time and energy during the day, eradicates appetite and cravings, allows me to actually eat to satiety, all while supporting a healthy, slim physique!

THE SCIENCE OF FASTING

Fasting induces hormonal changes in the body which sustain energy, protect protein stores, and moderate insulin release. In order to understand the benefits of intermittent fasting, and why you will be neither hungry nor lethargic (I promise!), let's look at what happens on a cellular level during a fast. Things are about to get sciency and real. If you couldn't care less about the specifics, feel free to skip ahead. But if you're a *Give-Me-Information-I-Must-Understand-WHY* sort (like me), you may find this interesting.

WHAT HAPPENS WHEN YOU EAT

Before understanding what happens during fasting, let's first establish what happens during eating… since we seem to be more familiar with that one.

Food is composed of *protein, fat,* and *carbohydrates.* Protein is used for repair and structure in the body. Fat is used for growth, repair, and energy, with excess stored in fat cells. Carbohydrates are essentially just used for energy, and are a bit more complicated. They are first converted into *glucose* for energy in the blood stream, which is known as "blood sugar." Because excess sugar is toxic to the body, the pancreas releases the storage hormone *insulin* to shuttle any extra glucose into the liver and muscles to be stored as *glycogen*. These stores, however, are limited: the average person can store around 15 grams per pound of body weight of glycogen. So if the glycogen reserves are full (which is quite often the case in our sugary, floury, carby society), the leftovers are stored as fat.

Oh, and insulin shuts off fat burning.

As such, the typical carb-fueled eating pattern of today, with sugary food available 24/7, encourages the body to wait around for glucose from meals, while storing fat for a "starving" period that may never come. This leads to fluctuating and reduced energy levels, as you live from carb to carb, rather than using fat stores. Such a state encourages weight gain, obesity, and diabetes.

WHAT HAPPENS WHEN YOU FAST

During fasting, the body shifts from using glucose (sugar from carbohydrates) as a primary fuel source, to *fatty acids*. This happens by increased *lipolysis,* the break down of stored fat in your white adipose tissue (the physical stuff on your body) into free fatty acids and glycerol in the blood stream. These released fatty acids can then be used for energy, growth, and repair. If they aren't ultimately used, they are mostly re-esterified (restored) as fat on your body.

Here's how it goes down.

Within 12 hours of fasting (12 hours since your last meal), the amount of fatty acids in the blood stream begins to increase (thanks to the lipolysis process discussed above). Previously stored body fat which *was* inertly sitting on your body now floats around in the bloodstream, ready for instant use! Between 18 and 24 hours of fasting, the amount of freed-up fatty acids substantially increases. By 72 hours of fasting, free fatty acids peak and plateau. At this point, there are 200-300x the amount of fatty acids in your bloodstream than when you last ate. Fat burning mode much? (**Note:** I'm just relaying the fasting timeline here, not recommending you jump on a 3 day fast. That would qualify as straight-up "fasting" rather than "intermittent fasting.")

In fact, the body releases almost *twice* as much fat from storage into the blood stream when fasting than needed for the *resting metabolic rate*: the amount of energy required to sustain vital body functions if you did nothing but simply exist. While people worry about a lack of energy when fasting, fasting actually *over-saturates* the body with energy through these increased fatty acid levels. And while the majority of the unused fatty acids are restored in white adipose tissue, this process does not account for *all* of the extra fatty acids released. Muscles and other tissues increase their fat storage capabilities when fasted, so extra fatty acids may be stored there, or used in other biosynthetic and metabolic pathways.

In simpler terms, the body "jumps the gun" when fasting by pulling *way too much* body fat out of its stored state to be used for energy. Not all of the unused freed-up body fat goes back to the fat stores you can "see" again. Instead, fasting encourages other processes and organs in the body to begin using and storing fat. With fasting, fat is no longer sitting around as a backup plan for the body: it now *is* the plan. How awesome is that?

This increase in fatty acid release, use, and storage is akin to the commonly heralded "fat burning mode." The body becomes super efficient at cycling fat, using it at any place, any time. Tissues throughout the entire body become more efficient at using fat for fuel. Unlike the non-fasted, carb-fed (glucose) state, when fat is tightly locked away for "special occasions," fasting encourages quick and easy use of fat for energy and other needs. The body no longer hesitates to release fat from storage. You become a "fat burning machine," including when exercising. (See Chapter 19: *Exercise, IF Style* for more on that!)

With the increase in free fatty acids comes a corresponding decrease in *glucose oxidation*. The body's glucose needs fall by around 44%. That's right: you won't "need" as much sugar! Muscle glycogen stores (the glucose stored in muscle) is particularly preserved while fasting, and can even *increase* by 10%. These "mystery carbs" can come from the liver, which can produce glucose from amino acids and glycerol through a process called *gluconeogenesis*.

The change in glucoregulatory hormones when fasting is supported by a fall in *insulin* levels and increased *insulin sensitivity*, effectively lowering, stabilizing, and discouraging fluctuations of blood sugar. This not only supports fat burning: it also means you'll be just fine with less carbs than before. And since it takes about 2 days of resumed "normal" feeding to reverse this positive effect, one meal with carbs probably won't make your body immediately switch back to preferring sugar and preserving fat for fuel. This partly explains why fasting on a cyclical daily basis (à la intermittent fasting) may let you "get away with" more carbs than you could before.

KETOSIS

In addition to upregulated fat and downregulated glucose use, the liver also begins producing *ketones* from fatty acids as a supplemental source of energy. Ketones are a very efficient and clean source of energy for the brain. They're kind of awesome all around. The brain actually runs more efficiently when utilizing ketones, rather than just glucose. Ketones are also neuro-protective for the brain. *Ketosis* refers to the body's elevated use of ketones for fuel, rather than sugar (which would be the state of *glycolysis*). In comparison to low fat diets, ketogenic diets are marked by increased adherence, greater weight loss from fat, and improved cholesterol levels. Full blown ketogenic diets are used to reduce seizure rates in epileptic patients, reduce tremors in Parkinson's disease, regain memory in Alzheimer's patients, help control blood sugar in diabetes, and even fight cancer. Check out *Keto Clarity: Your Definitive Guide to the Benefits of a Low-Carb, High-Fat Diet* by Jimmy Moore for an in-depth look at all the amazing benefits of a strict ketogenic diet.

Note: Ketosis is a healthy, regulated metabolic state, not to be confused with *ketoacidosis*. Ketoacidosis is an abnormal, dangerous diabetic state of ketosis which can potentially occur in diabetics (typically Type 1), who lack insulin to regulate the state. It does not occur in insulin-producing individuals.

SO WHAT DOES IT ALL MEAN?

To summarize all this fasting madness, short-term fasting forces the body into a highly sustainable fat burning mode saturated in energy, irony of "fasting" aside. The entire body becomes excellent at using fat for energy, supplemented by ketones, while glucose needs drop. Blood sugar levels lower and stabilize, and the body becomes quite insulin sensitive. The fasted state is one of ample energy, health, and vitality.

CHAPTER THIRTEEN

HOW TO DO INTERMITTENT FASTING

There are many different patterns of intermittent fasting (IF) you can try. The key thing to remember is that you are focusing on restricting the *hours* you eat, not necessarily the *amount of food* you eat (although you may find this happens naturally). These "eating windows," and how much you eat during them, vary quite a bit. You can jump all in with a daily fast, switch it up a few days a week, or just fast "here and there" whenever you're so inclined. Keep in mind that the beneficial metabolic changes from fasting typically begin 12 hours or so after your last meal, with the "golden hour" (maximum return on investment, fat burning wise) occurring 16-24 hours or so after your last meal.

Here are some common patterns in the intermittent fasting world.

1. Daily Time Window Fast
Implementing a regulated time window is a good technique if you're new to the intermittent fasting world. In this popular approach, you eat each day during a set "window" of

your choosing. The eating window is usually around 6-10 hours or so, and encompasses the entire amount of calories and nutrients for the day. For example, you might eat from 8:00am-4:00pm, 12:00pm-6:00pm, 5:00pm-12:00am, or something similar. It's really up to you! Just pick a window, and try to keep it consistent each day.

Martin Berkhan's popular *Leangains* protocol (http://www.leangains.com) advocates a consistent 16/8 pattern, in which you fast for 16 hours, and then eat during an 8 hour window. *Leangains* also has specific food macronutrient patterns and supplements, and is tailored towards bodybuilders.

2. Daily Meal-Based Fast
In this intermittent fasting approach, you eat certain meals each day, rather than during a certain time frame. For example, you could eat breakfast and lunch, lunch and dinner, or only dinner. The meal eating window encompasses the entire amount of calories and nutrients for the day.

The Warrior Diet by Ori Hofmekle is an example of this approach: he advocates fasting during the day and feasting each night. This is what I have been doing ever since reading Rusty Moore's post *Lose Body Fat By Eating Just One Meal Per Day?* (http://www.fitnessblackbook.com/dieting_for_fat_loss/lose-body-fat-by-eating-just-one-meal-per-day/) in 2011. I eat dinner each night (whenever it happens to occur based on hunger or social situations), and then freely munch until bed.

3. Weekly Fast
If you choose a structured weekly fast, you will eat "normally" most days, but throw in some intermittent fasting a few days per week. This could be a smaller 16 hour-ish fast, or longer 24 hour one. Since you're not fasting daily, you don't need to focus on getting a day's worth of calories, and can just eat a normal meal if you desire. (However, you can certainly "feast" and still see benefits).

Brad Pilon's *Eat Stop Eat* (http://www.bradpilon.com) is a good example of this approach. He advocates a weekly or biweekly complete 24 hour fast, broken with a normal sized meal.

4. The Random Fast
Of course, you don't have to stick to any certain protocol! You can always simply eat when hungry, while throwing in an elongated fast here and there. The nice thing about having some fasting under your belt, is knowing you can pull it out of your proverbial pocket whenever you feel like it!

Chapter Fourteen

Tips For Intermittent Fasting

While the thought of *not* eating for a bit may seem scary, intermittent fasting becomes super easy, super quick! Fasting becomes a time when you're just... *not hungry*. Check out these tips to calm your fears and ease the transition!

1. Arm Yourself With Knowledge
Know that you will NOT die if you don't eat for a few hours. Thinking what you're doing is harmful or antagonistic will make fasting a huge hurdle in your mind. Stress helps nothing. Read articles and do research (like the rest of this book, for example!) to understand what's actually happening in your body during a fast.

2. Feast Before
Don't commence your fast in a hungry state. If you're doing the common evening hours or dinner protocol like me, consider eating *a lot* the night before starting. Channel the *"I'm so stuffed I could never eat again!"* feeling. That way, you won't even be hungry for a substantial part of the first

fasting day. Once you've got a day under your belt, you'll be more motivated for day 2, and the days to follow. I find that if I can do something for a day, I can do it many days!

3. Fill Your Schedule
Keep your schedule busy during the fasting window. If you've constantly got something to do, you won't be as likely to encounter the all-too-common boredom munchies.

4. Stay Active
Keep on moving! Physical activity upregulates lipolysis and fat burning. It pairs well with fasting, while actually enhancing it! If you simply lie around in a melodramatically lethargic *"I'm fasting"* mindset, it will only make things more difficult, rather than help matters.

5. Caffeine
Caffeine is your friend, at least in the beginning. Caffeine blunts appetite and increases lipolysis. Drink tea and coffee during the fast; just don't load them with cream and sugar.

6. Make Sleep Your Friend
Sleep is not only your health friend in general - it also totally counts towards your fasting window. It's hard to be hungry when you're asleep! Consider timing your sleep to give you a sort of "head start." For example, if you've picked an evening feeding window, you could have a big, early dinner the night before fasting. By the time you wake up the next morning, you'll be significantly into your fast already! Definitely don't begin your fasting adventures when you know you'll be sleep deprived, which will make everything unnecessarily difficult.

7. Consider Starting Slow
You can always try just skipping breakfast here and there for starters, and then gradually increase consistency or the fasting window time.

8. Try Just 3 Days
Committing to an IF pattern for just 3 days will probably get

you hooked. If you can make it to day 3 (which you can!), chances are you'll be in LOVE with intermittent fasting by that point, and will desire to continue it. When I first started intermittent fasting, I committed to a week. That was over 3 years ago, and I haven't stopped!

9. Consider Going Low Carb Or Paleo First
Adopting a low carb or Paleo diet is another way to make your body super efficient at fat burning. If you're already low carb and "fat adapted," fasting will likely be a breeze from the get-go.

10. See IF As A Learning Experiment, Rather Than A "Test"
When you first start intermittent fasting, don't look at it as a pass or fail test; rather, look at intermittent fasting as a way to experience something *new*. To see how a different meal pattern feels. To try something different! Instead of thinking, *"I will do this for a week, otherwise it was pointless,"* think, *"I will do this for a week, and then I will know how it feels."*

Chapter Fifteen

Intermittent Fasting Benefits

People often assume fasting is detrimental to health, when in reality it is quite the opposite. Check out these awesome health and lifestyle benefits which come from adding a bit of fasting to your life!

INTERMITTENT FASTING HEALTH BENEFITS

1. Increased Lifespan
Scientific studies consistently correlate intermittent fasting with increased lifespan. While the exact mechanisms are unknown, the anti-aging benefits of fasting may stem from increased insulin sensitivity and the downregulation of insulin and insulin-like peptides. Fasting also counteracts aging's effects on genes by decreasing oxidative stress while strengthening immunity and energy metabolism. In fact, yeast cells were up to 1000 times more protected against oxidative stress when fasted! Similar results were found in mice.

2. Stress Resistance
Like exercise, fasting acts as a mild, beneficial stressor to the body, conditioning cells to resist future stress.

3. Autophagy
Fasting promotes autophagy, a sort of clean-up process where the body recycles old, damaged, and unused proteins. Autophagy is required for cells to survive. Like a "cleanse" on the cellular level, autophagy discourages the accumulation of toxins which can lead to frailty and atrophy (a wasting away of cells), while supporting muscle mass. Autophagy also slows down the aging process and protects against age-related diseases. In fact, aging is directly correlated to decreased rates of autophagy in the body.

4. Immune Support/ Disease Resistance
Before my intermittent fasting days, colds were "normal." Intermittent fasting, however, works wonders for the immune system, and now I rarely get sick. Intermittent fasting supports the immune system by discouraging inflammatory responses, reducing oxidative damage, and increasing stress resistance. In fact, studies show intermittent fasting literally changes gene expressions on a cellular level, regulating inflammatory responses (which is quite different from popping a pill to calm inflammation). Fasting also increases phagocytosis of white blood cells: the process by which they "eat" and expunge bacteria and other toxins. During a fast, the liver stores less fat, potentially protecting it against insulin resistance-induced liver diseases, like non-alcoholic fatty liver disease. Intermittent fasting's disease resistance benefits even extend to the brain, protecting against neurodegenerative diseases such as Alzheimer's, Parkinson's disease, Huntington's disease, and stroke.

5. Cancer Prevention
Studies show intermittent fasting reduces cancer risk and cell proliferation rates. Furthermore, this beneficial fasting effect works selectively on cancerous cells, encouraging growth of normal cells and protecting them from oxidative stress, while retarding growth of cancerous ones *without* shielding them from oxidative stress. A 2009 review of 10 different patient

studies published in *Aging* found fasting improved the nasty side effects of chemotherapy, reducing fatigue and weakness, while completely eliminating vomiting and diarrhea. In fact, 2-3 weeks of alternate day fasting pre-chemotherapy has been shown to "improve outcomes in cancer chemotherapy, decreasing morbidity and raising cure rates."

6. Increased Insulin Sensitivity

Intermittent fasting reduces fasting insulin and discourages insulin resistance and the many problems stemming from such, including metabolic syndrome, obesity, and diabetes. Benefits of increased insulin sensitivity include enhanced nutrition partitioning, decreased appetite, lowered cholesterol, and weight loss.

7. Human Growth Hormone Release

You'd think intermittent fasting would stunt growth, but fasting actually encourages human growth hormone (HGH) release, a hormone which stimulates cell reproduction and regeneration. As we age, HGH release declines. Since consuming food blocks HGH release, fasting functions like a double negative in removing the inhibition of HGH. Furthermore, enhanced HGH secretion during fasting encourages lipolysis and fat burning.

8. Enhanced Brain Function

Intermittent Fasting provides a constant stream of fatty acids to fuel the central nervous system, keeping your brain alert and active. Fasting also encourages the use of ketones, an incredibly efficient source of fuel for the brain. Ketones promote memory and learning, while slowing neurological disease processes. The brain also functions better when supplemented with ketones, rather than when utilizing glucose alone. Intermittent fasting also increases alertness by upregulating norepinephrine, a neurotransmitter which increases vigilant concentration. The upregulation of the central nervous system has been cited as a potential reason for the seemingly contradictory idea of increased resting energy expenditure while fasting.

Intermittent fasting also provides anti-aging benefits to the brain and protects it from metabolic and oxidative stress.

It promotes neurogenesis (the production of new neurons in the brain) as well as neuroplasticity (change and adaptation within the brain which decreases with age). Fasting increases "brain-derived neurotrophic factor," which aids brain neurons in resisting dysfunction and degeneration. Intermittent fasting also promotes autophagy, the cellular "cleanup" discussed above, within the brain.

9. Mood
Studies have shown meal patterns influence mood in general. Fasting specifically encourages a good mood by raising norepinephrine and dopamine levels. Intermittent fasting also controls blood sugar levels and insulin, eradicating feelings of being "hangry" - that angry feeling you get when blood sugar levels drop and you don't want to talk to anyone because you MUST EAT SOMETHING NOW. A 2014 study looking at non-diabetic adults found fluctuating blood sugar levels were actually associated with anger: high blood sugar levels made it difficult to control anger. The study even suggested anger may be a risk factor for diabetes.

10. Enhanced Exercise
Contrary to common belief, fasting does *not* negatively affect exercise. Fasted exercise actually maximizes fat oxidation, increases muscular oxidative capacity, and prevents blood sugar crashes and the "hitting the wall" feeling which typically occur from exercise in the fed state. Fasted exercise also *increases* muscle protein synthesis. If you want to maximize fat burning, fasted exercise is the way to go, since the entire body, including muscle, relies primarily on fatty acids while fasted.

INTERMITTENT FASTING LIFE BENEFITS

1. More Time
You'd be surprised how much time you "gain" when you don't have to constantly interrupt your routine for food. Intermittent fasting gives you a beautiful lengthy time window of opportunity without distraction. When I wake up, I can immediately jump into my day, which goes interrupted

until dinner. Oh, and there's less dishes to wash as well!

2. Save Money
Although you may be consuming the same amount of calories as before, intermittent fasting tends to save you money. For me, prepping one meal per day is much more efficient than making many meals throughout the day. You also won't be constantly buying random snacks, which add up quickly.

3. Easy Travel
Intermittent fasting makes diet choices while traveling super easy. *"What will I eat at the airport?"* or *"What will I eat on the road trip?"* are no longer issues! Plus, you get a little more leeway and "protection" when you *do* eat at your final destination, as intermittent fasting encourages nutrient partitioning and discourages fat gain.

4. Increased Stamina
Since intermittent fasting is fueled by (essentially) unlimited fatty acids from stored body fat, your stamina substantially increases. Once in the fasted state, you feel like you can just keep going forever! Gone is the fear of running out of energy, "hitting the wall," and becoming tired. *You just know you can do it.*

5. Admiration
While many people may write you off as crazy, some will admire your "incredible" self control, wishing they could do the same. Yes it's an ego boost, but these feelings of awe can make you feel pretty good. (This is tinged by irony, given the relative ease of implementing intermittent fasting. See Chapter 16: *Why Intermittent Fasting Is Easy* for more on that.)

6. Increased Willpower
Speaking of willpower, intermittent fasting requires very little willpower because it's so easy to do. Still, sticking to it reiterates feelings of self control and goal accomplishment. Studies have shown that achieving control and success in one area (like diet) strengthens your "willpower" muscle, encouraging increased willpower in other areas of your life!

In fact, rats put on fasting protocols were more likely to break their cocaine addictions!

7. Avoid "Ego Depletion"
With intermittent fasting, you make substantially less food decisions over the course of the day, saving you from "decision fatigue" or "ego depletion." Studies show that the very act of making decisions actually drains energy reserves, and decreases your "decision making ability." As a 2007 review in *Social and Personality Psychology Compass* 1 notes, "After making many choices, the chooser is less able to engage in good self control, suggesting that making choices exhausts the self over time." While it may seem silly to apply this concept to something as "simple" as meals, all those constant food choices throughout the day really add up! In a typical eating pattern, you must choose when *and* what to eat 3-6 times per day. That's a lot of choices! With intermittent fasting, I personally choose what to eat once per day. (Sometimes I don't even make that choice, if I've already planned it out.) I love not thinking about food until dinner, which leaves an abundance of brain power to use elsewhere, like writing this book for example! This also means when it comes time to eat, you'll more likely make good food choices! {cough} Paleo. {cough}

8. Understand Appetite Vs. Hunger
Intermittent fasting gives you clarity of mind concerning whimsy appetite in contrast to actual hunger. With fasting, you will know when you *want* something versus when you *need* something. It's quite empowering and revolutionary. When you *do* experience cravings (like when walking by the cake mix section in the grocery store - curse you Funfetti!), you can accurately assess the situation. You can calmly tell the craving, *"You have no power over me!" Labyrinth* style.

9. Lose The "Hungry" Fear
Intermittent fasting kills the fear of a ravenous appetite. In fact, the longer you go into a fast, the *less* hungry you often become. You no longer have to worry about planning snacks or when you're going to eat. You know you can go a substantial amount of time without food, and come out just

dandy (and healthy) on the other end.

10. Enjoy Food Without Guilt Or Restriction
Intermittent fasting is truly the solution to effortless weight loss without feelings of deprivation or restriction. You can eat all you want and still burn fat, including those pesky "stubborn" areas. You can finally eat without a smidge of guilt! It's a fabulous feeling to indulge, is it not?

Chapter Sixteen

Why Intermittent Fasting Is Easy

Back in my e*at-3-meals-plus-snacks-in-between-days,* I always seemed to be hungry, or at least fantasizing about my next meal. It seemed that once I began eating on any given day, I simply wanted to keep munching *all* day. Know the feeling? Intermittent fasting is quite liberating because it *eradicates all food cravings* for the majority of the day. As long as you are consuming adequate nutrients, intermittent fasting is a natural and healthy way of eating. It's super easy, thanks to a physical loss of appetite, psychological loss of cravings, increased willpower, and effortless results. (It's no wonder that studies consistently find high compliance rates for patients on fasting protocols.) If you want to know the sciency mechanisms at play here, read on!

PHYSICAL LOSS OF APPETITE

Studies consistently find a loss of appetite in patients following fasting protocols. While normal dieting (often in the form of calorie restriction) increases hunger, fasting blunts hunger. As a 2007 article in *The Proceedings of the Nutrition Society* notes, "Dieting or restrained eating generally increase the likelihood of food craving, while fasting makes craving, like hunger, diminish."

Consider a fascinating 1990 Swedish study comparing hunger and craving levels when people "diet" versus when they "fast." Two groups of obese patients (one dieting via calorie restriction, the other dieting via fasting) recorded their appetite and cravings over a 3 week treatment period. They were shown pictures of food to evaluate their hunger and craving levels. By the end of the trial, the "dieting" group experienced very minimal changes in hunger and cravings: they were still hankering for food. The fasting group, however, lost *all* reactivity to food stimuli, with hunger and craving reactions measured almost zero! The study concluded that hunger and cravings remain constant with calorie restriction diets, while hunger and cravings decrease with fasting diets. (The "zero reactivity" to food stimuli is definitely what fasting feels like to me. I see people eating lunch and I'm like, *"Hmm that looks nice... don't care!"*)

A more recent 2010 *University of Illinois* study examined the body's adaptations to fasting to see how such changes affect weight loss. Noting the difficulties of common calorie restriction, which requires *constant* food limitation, the study proposed an "alternate day modified fast" (ADMF) approach. Patients alternated fasting days of restricted food intake (25% of baseline needs) from 12:00-2:00pm, with ad libitum feeding days. The patients followed a 4 week controlled phase implementing the ADMF with all meals provided, followed by another 4 week period of ADMF, this time implementing the entire regime themselves. Physical activity was maintained throughout the trial.

The patients recorded their levels of hunger and satisfaction. While they reported being hungry the first week, hunger decreased by the second week and remained low throughout the rest of the trial (similar to the Swedish study previously discussed). Levels of satisfaction, however, consistently *increased!* As for weight loss, the patients consistently lost weight, even with ad libitum feeding days when they ate *all they wanted*, and even when implementing the protocol themselves.

The study also expected to find phagia (increased appetite) on the days the patients could eat normally, hypothesizing that the patients would "make up for" the fast by overeating on their feast day by 25%. But they didn't. The patients actually ate 5-10% *less* than their "required" energy levels on their free days!

These results show that, unlike calorie restriction, adopting a fasting pattern of eating blunts hunger and increases satisfaction, while sustaining weight loss. Furthermore, fasting does *not* encourage an inevitably ravenous appetite once one resumes eating. The study concluded that people "quickly adapt to ADMF," with the degree and rate of weight loss affected by how many and what type of calories are consumed, along with physical activity.

WHY THE LOSS OF APPETITE?

While studies like the ones discussed consistently find a loss of appetite when fasting, why does this loss of appetite occur? The main reasons involve body fuel changes, stabilized blood sugar, increased insulin sensitivity, and cellular and hormonal adaptation.

Let's look at each of these.

1. Fuel Changes

Fasting ramps up *lipolysis*, increasing the amount of fatty acids in the blood stream. This primes the body for the long haul, giving it access to a sustainable energy supply from stored body fat, unlike the limited and wavering carbohydrate stores it's likely accustomed to. Unless you're at a dangerously low body weight, you have enough fuel reserves (body fat) to sustain you for *quite* a substantial amount of time. In fact, a 145 lb person with 18% body fat (a BMI considered "underweight") has enough stored fat to walk approximately 1000 miles! With the "assurance" of fuel in the fasted state, appetite for food (energy) decreases. In simpler terms, fasting decreases hunger and appetite because it fills you with energy from *within* you, rather than from food. It's like when people say, *"You always had it in you!"*... except you did, quite literally.

2. Stabilized Blood Sugar

The counterpart to the use of fatty acids for fuel is a decreased reliance on sugar. Sugar stores (glucose in the form of glycogen) are a fleeting thing, determined by your last meal or snack. Your glycogen stores are limited to around 15g per pound of body weight, which is why you can't stock up on carbs for the long haul. Fasting drastically reduces the body's need for glucose, switching instead to fat. Gone are the hunger signals instigated by low blood sugar a few hours (or less) after your last meal.

3. Increased Insulin Sensitivity
With the increase of fatty acids and decrease of glucose comes a lowered need for insulin. Elevated insulin levels increase hunger and fat storage, while lowered insulin levels reduce appetite and promote fat burning. If you're cells become desensitized to insulin (as promoted by constantly eating carbs), then insulin cannot properly transport nutrients into your body's cells, and stores it as fat instead. By encouraging insulin sensitivity, fasting teaches your body to properly utilize and store nutrients. Since your cells are being adequately energized, you have less appetite!

4. Cellular And Hormonal Changes
Fasting also encourages cellular and hormonal adaptations which reduce appetite. Cells in the body have inherent circadian rhythms which adapt to temporal feeding patterns. This is why the typical person becomes hungry at breakfast, lunch, and dinner. If you adopt a new consistent pattern of eating, your body's "hungry" signals adapt to match on a cellular level. (For me, I literally only get hungry around dinner time.) Rodent studies also show that periods of intermittent fasting upregulate *leptin*, a hormone which induces feelings of satiety, upon re-feeding. While leptin upregulation *typically* occurs from gaining adipose tissue, fasting somehow has a similar effect on leptin levels. This means when you *do* eat in an intermittent fasting protocol, you may become "fuller" sooner, and stay satiated for longer.

PSYCHOLOGICAL LOSS OF CRAVINGS

In addition to the discussed "physical" appetite adjustments (fuel changes, stabilized blood sugar, insulin sensitivity, and cellular adaptations), fasting also eliminates psychological cravings by eradicating *feelings of deprivation* and *allowing satiety*, which are key in maintaining a diet lifestyle. In my calorie counting diet days, I fretted nonstop about portion sizes, "servings," and of course calories. With a fasting regime, I can eat *all I want* at night and feel satiated, while still maintaining a low body fat percentage.

This is quite unlike a "dieting" mindset, which increases food cravings. One study analyzed 129 women's food craving records over a one week period. Some were dieting, some were "watching their weight," and some were non-dieters. Of the nearly 400 cravings reported, the "dieters" featured substantially more cravings than the "non-dieters." (The "watchers" fell in between.) The study concluded a link between dieting and food cravings, especially since mood, situations, and time between eating were not distinguishing factors.

Fascinatingly, cravings associated with the dieting mindset do not necessarily result from the actual amount of calories consumed or any actual deficiency, as one might assume. Rather, the restrictive mindset and lack of satiation in the typical dieting protocol can instigate feelings of "perceived deprivation." A study on dieting individuals found that this perceived deprivation within a dieter's mind does not actually correlate to actual deprivation or calorie intake, but instead comes from *psychological unfulfillment*. It concluded that dieters "may experience a sense of deprivation not because they are eating less than they *need* but because they are eating less than they *want*." Since intermittent fasting allows one to eat to satiety, it prevents the psychological feelings of deprivation which create cravings in the typical dieting scenario.

INCREASED WILLPOWER

"Wow, you must have a lot of willpower!" people often exclaim when they learn of my fasting habits. I used to tell them I actually have *no* willpower, since it's "all or none" for me. Then I read Charles Duhigg's *The Power of Habit* and realized intermittent fasting may *literally* be less taxing on willpower.

Psychology professor Mark Muraven tested the limits of willpower by presenting students with bowls of radishes and cookies. Some were told to only eat the cookies, others just the radishes. They were then given a puzzle to finish, unaware it was actually impossible (which I find pretty hysterical). The "radish students" easily gave up, while the "cookie students" worked much longer on the puzzle. Presumably, the students who had "exerted" some of their willpower by ignoring the cookies, had less willpower remaining to work on the puzzle. Muraven notes that over 200 studies on willpower have found this same idea: "Willpower isn't just a skill. It's a muscle, like the muscles in your arms or legs, and it gets tired as it works harder, so there's less power left over for other things."

A typical diet *overwhelmingly drains willpower.* You must constantly restrict meals, refuse snacks, and resist food you want to eat. Eating is always an option, and always a temptation. Intermittent fasting is completely different. It eradicates appetite and cravings, so you no longer drain willpower resources. It's like the equivalent of eating while sleeping or playing a sport - simply not on your mind. Nor do you tempt willpower when you *do* finally eat, since you can eat all you wish!

In fact, fasting doesn't just sustain willpower, it may even increase it! A 2006 series of three willpower studies performed by Australian researchers Megan Oaten and Ken Cheng found that exhibiting willpower in one area of life (like dieting) increased willpower in other areas of life (like TV watching and smoking addictions). As a 2006 *Journal of Personality* study says, "Regular exercises in self-regulation can produce broad improvements in self-regulation (like strengthening a muscle), making people less vulnerable to ego depletion." This increased willpower from fasting may also explain why a 2010 study actually found that *fasting helped rats break cocaine addictions!* That one kind of seals the deal for me.

EFFORTLESS RESULTS

A final reason intermittent fasting is incredibly easy to maintain is because it eliminates the hunger, cravings, and guilt of calorie restriction, while still being just as effective. With intermittent fasting, you will never count calories, or weigh and measure food again! You can eat a king's feast (especially if Paleo), yet consume less than you would consciously dieting. You don't even have to concentrate on "exercise" for fat burning to take place, and weight loss to occur! Better yet, maintenance of your new low weight becomes second nature rather than a chore. As you finally see progress in your goals without pain and deprivation, motivation soars. Intermittent fasting truly is effortlessly easy.

CHAPTER SEVENTEEN

THE MYTHS OF METABOLISM

If you're considering intermittent fasting, you might be a little nervous about your "metabolism" - a controlling concept shrouded in mystery. You may think this vague metabolism will irrecoverably slow down and enter "starvation mode" if you eat too few calories (below 1200!), or not every few hours. To reassure you, let's look at the science of the metabolism to understand the genesis of these myths, as such they are.

Note: I will be using the "calorie" terminology in discussing the metabolism, as a basic way to measure the amount of energy taken in via food in comparison to the amount of energy utilized (or "burned") by the body. I do, however, believe that both "metabolism" and "calories" are very broad terms for very complicated processes, and that fat burning and storage involves much more than a simple "calories in vs. calories out" approach. See *In Consideration of Calories* for more on that.

WHAT IS THE METABOLISM?

The "metabolism" is a poorly misunderstood concept, especially given how casually it's thrown around in the diet world. People often think of the metabolism as a fixed amount of "calories" a person burns per day. But it's not that simple. (Is it ever?) The word "metabolism" comes from the Greek word metabolē, which translates to "change." And indeed, the metabolism is not some fixed number of calories - it is always in flux.

It's a complicated matter, but let's take a stab at it! A person's *"daily metabolic rate"* or *"total metabolism"* for a day is determined by three basic things: *the basal metabolic rate* (BMR), the *thermic effect of food*, and the *physical activity energy expenditure* for that day. We'll break these down one by one, and shed light on their associated myths.

1. BASAL METABOLIC RATE (BMR)

The "basal metabolic rate" refers to the amount of energy required to sustain all the vital organs (including ventilation, blood circulation, and temperature regulation) at rest for a day. In other words, it is the amount of "calories" required if you literally did *nothing* for an entire day, in a calm, temperate environment, since even stimulating the nervous system affects this rate. (So you couldn't even think about exciting things: your BMR is devoid of emotion!)

Formulas abound to calculate a person's BMR. The most common and basic ones use height, weight, age, and gender. This notably does not account for body composition, as muscle burns more calories than fat. Two people could be the same height, weight, age, and gender, but if one person has more muscle than the other, he or she will likely have a higher BMR.

> **The Myth:** *You won't lose weight if you eat too few calories, or go too long without eating, because your BMR falls to compensate.*

This myth comes from a spark of truth, but brings it to the *entirely* wrong conclusion. Yes, your BMR *does* adjust based on a consistent calorie intake. But no, it will not stop weight loss, nor is the BMR's adjustment irreversible or even a "bad thing." Let's look at the effects of both calorie restriction and fasting on BMR to understand why.

1. Calorie Restriction And Basal Metabolic Rate

If you follow a calorie restricted diet for an extended period of time, your BMR will likely lower to compensate. The body "wants" to live, and will make metabolic changes to promote long-term survival. If you're consistently consuming too little energy, the body will slow down the amount of energy it "requires." It's smart like that. However, this change does not stop weight loss or fat burning. It won't kill you. And it won't be stuck there for ever. (Remember "metabolism" means "change.") When a person implements steady calorie restriction, the metabolism adjusts to cover the difference. But assuming the calorie restriction is below the amount of calories required for that day, the person will still lose weight - just at a slower pace than if the metabolism *hadn't* adjusted for the deficit.

Take for instance an extensive 2006 study at a Louisiana research center which looked at the effects of 6 months of calorie restriction in healthy, overweight (but not obese) men and women. The study included 4 groups: a control group on a maintenance diet, a 25% calorie restricted diet group, a 25% calorie restricted diet and exercise group (12.5% from calorie restriction, 12.5% from exercise), and a very low calorie group at 890 calories (who assumed a maintenance diet after losing 15% of their weight). While the study found a substantial decrease in metabolic rate in all the calorie restricted patients, *they still all lost weight throughout the trial.* At no point did weight loss stop. Also, the reduced metabolic rate occurred within 3 months, but did not lower after that.

The takeaway? Not getting "enough" calories will not stop your weight loss: you simply will burn less fat than if your BMR hadn't lowered to compensate. Weight loss may plateau from the metabolism "dropping" if one loses enough weight so that their deficit is no longer a "deficit" for their new weight. For example, say you restrict your diet to a rate which cannot sustain your present weight, but *could* sustain your body at a lower weight (since the less you weigh, the less calories you require). Once your body reaches that lower weight, you would then need to further lower calories to continue weight loss.

Oh, and while we're on the subject, a slowed down metabolism reduces body temperature, fasting insulin levels, and DNA damage. All of these factors increase longevity. Yep, a "slower metabolism" could actually mean you live longer. Such irony.

2. Fasting And Basal Metabolic Rate

While the *calorie-restriction-slowing-metabolism* myth bears some credence (since one's BMR does indeed adjust to calorie restriction), the *meal-frequency-slowing-metabolism* myth is just plain false. As long as you are consuming adequate energy and nutrients in total each day (meaning you are not calorie restricted), your BMR will *not* slow down in response to meal frequency. Studies on meal frequency and metabolism consistently find no metabolic adjustment to reduced meal timing. As noted in the 1997 *British Journal of Nutrition*, "Studies using whole-body calorimetry and doubly-labelled water to assess total 24 h energy expenditure find no difference between nibbling and gorging." In fact, the metabolic rate can potentially *increase* while fasting. A 2000 *American Journal of Nutrition* study analyzing the basal metabolic rate in healthy lean individuals at various stages of fasting (between 1-84 hours), found their BMR increased throughout the *entire* trial.

To reiterate, calorie restriction, not meal frequency, is what "slows down" the BMR and reduces the rate of weight loss. Intermittent fasting, if consuming adequate calories in the eating window, does *not* negatively affect one's BMR. And to make things even more complicated (just because we can!), when calorie restriction is coupled with fasting, it may not even lower BMR! The aforementioned 2006 Louisiana study suggested that "energy deficit rather than calorie restriction itself (drives) the decrease in energy expenditure." Since fasting provides ample energy via fat metabolism, calorie restriction may be "safer" when fasting than when practiced throughout the day. Fasting upregulates hormones which prevent energy deficit (via fat and ketone use), so a reduced BMR may not occur, even when in a deficit.

The Myth: *Dieting permanently damages your metabolism. You'll gain all the weight back when you stop, and then some.*

This is another metabolism myth based in truth, but taken to a faulty conclusion. Yes, calorie restriction and weight loss (with no compensatory muscle gain) lower the basal metabolic rate. However, a lower body weight correlates to a lower metabolism: if there's less "of" you, there's less energy needed to *sustain* you. (Remember the basic formula for BMR includes gender, height, age, and *weight*.) So if you lose 10 pounds from dieting, you may now have a lower metabolic rate compared to your formerly heavier self, but this is simply because your new weight equates to a lower metabolism. While perhaps permanent at that new weight, the change is not irreversible. If you revert to the increased amount of calories you were eating before, you'll likely go back to that higher weight and its correlated higher metabolism.

A study of women who achieved stable weight loss through calorie restriction concluded they had "metabolic rates *appropriate for* their body sizes." In other words, your metabolism may settle at a lower point from weight loss, but it won't be lower than it *should* be for the "new you."

2. THERMIC EFFECT OF FOOD

The "thermic effect of food" refers to the amount of energy (or "calories") required to digest and process food. Digestion is quite a taxing process, explaining why you may get tired after a big meal. (Hello post-Thanksgiving nap!) In general, the thermic effect of food (or "diet induced thermogenesis") is around 10% of calories consumed. The type of food consumed, however, affects the level of thermogenesis. Protein yields the highest thermic effect, with carbs coming in second. Fat is relatively benign, with barely any thermic effect. Eating protein therefore "burns more" (or on the flipside, counts as "less calories"), than eating the same amount of calories from carbs or fat.

The Myth: *You must eat constantly to speed up your metabolism.*

Since eating does temporarily "speed up the metabolism" due to food's thermic effect, we get the myth that you should *constantly* eat to speed up your metabolism. The thermic effect, however, is a *percentage* based on the amount and macronutrients of food consumed, not the frequency. This percentage does not change based on meal frequency or even calorie restriction. It doesn't matter if 10 minutes or 10 hours have passed since your last meal - the total thermic effect for the day will be a percentage of the total amount of calories consumed that day.

A study comparing 2 large meals versus 4 small meals in a day (both situations yielding the same total amount of calories), found *no difference* in the overall thermic effect for the day. Eating small meals throughout the day yields a steady, yet small thermic effect. Eating one or two meals in a restricted time window yields an isolated, yet substantially larger thermic effect. As long as you eat the same amount of calories for the day in both situations, the total thermic effect for the day will be the same.

For instance, if you eat 1800 calories throughout the day in 6 meals, you'd eat 300 calories per meal. That would be a 10% thermic effect of 30 calories per meal, for a total of 180 calories "burned" from eating. Now say you eat all 1800 calories in one meal. The thermic effect would be 10% of 1800, which is 180 calories "burned" from eating. See what happened? Either way you ultimately "raised" your metabolism the same amount over the course of the day. The difference is you either did it all at once, or slowly throughout the day. It's like if you went shopping all day and ended up with 6 outfits costing $180. Whether you bought them at different stores throughout the day, or all at once at a single store, the total cost would be the same.

That being said, if you eat MORE calories in the 6 meal scenario than the one meal scenario (which, speaking from experience, is pretty easy to do), then you would indeed "burn more calories" via the thermic effect from eating 6 meals than the one meal; however, you'd also be taking in and storing more calories with the 6 meals. So it's a moot point. You can't burn more fat overall by eating more. It's a silly concept.

3. PHYSICAL ACTIVITY ENERGY EXPENDITURE (EE)

"Physical activity energy expenditure" refers to the daily physical activity performed by a person, and thus the amount of energy needed for such activity as contributing to the overall "daily metabolic rate." This includes both conscious *volitional activity* (like sports and exercise), as well as *non-exercise activity thermogenesis* (NEAT), which is all the other movement you do in life, like fidgeting, walking from place to place, dancing, or even laughing!

The Myth: *Fasting makes you lethargic and low on energy, so you burn less calories.*

This myth actually involves the metabolic adaptations to fuel substrates rather than the "metabolism" per se. Fasting does not make you tired and lethargic, nor is it a state of energy depletion. Fasting encourages the body to utilize fats (from the plethora of stored body fat) as fuel, rather than limited glycogen (carb) stores. Because of this, the fasted state is alert and active. See Chapter 12: *What Is Intermittent Fasting* for an in-depth explanation of what happens during a fast, or Chapter 19: *Exercise, IF Style* to see how fasting actually increases energy expenditure and fat burning specifically during physical activity and exercise, and all in favor of one's "metabolism!"

SO WHAT DOES IT ALL MEAN?

Basically, you *really don't have to worry* about intermittent fasting damaging your metabolism. The "metabolism" slows down in relation to calorie restriction, not meal frequency. If adequate calories are consumed, intermittent fasting does not affect it. And even when the metabolism *does* slow down in response to calorie restriction or weight loss, you will *still* lose weight. (A lowered metabolism does not stop fat burning.) As for the thermic effect of food, it is a percentage of calories ingested overall, and does not change based on meal timing. You do not need to eat constantly to "raise your metabolism." Lastly, fasting does not make you tired and lethargic. On the contrary, it promotes ample energy and increased energy expenditure, as intermittent fasting primes the metabolism for fat burning, giving you much more bang for your buck!

CHAPTER EIGHTEEN

FAT BURNING, IF STYLE

The average person has enough stored fat to walk over 1,000 miles.

A typical lean person stores enough fat to survive over one month.

In some obese people, fat storage could support life for an entire year.

I don't know about you, but I find these facts staggering.

With so much body fat just *waiting* to be used, why is it seemingly so difficult to convince our bodies to actually *use* it? This question haunted my pre-fasting days, which were filled with calorie fixation. I'd monitor my intake, then run on the treadmill, watching the "calories burned" monitor increase at a frustratingly slow pace. I'd do endless crunches, "distracting" myself with the TV. (Hah!) 'Twas all in vain.

The key to burning fat is to change your body's "mindset." You've got to make it *want* to burn fat, rather than avoid doing such at all costs. Intermittent fasting is awesome because it effortlessly plunges you into the ever elusive "fat burning mode," switching your body from thinking, *"Only tap into body fat as a last resort!"* to *"Use fat for everything!"* When fasting, almost every movement you do and thought you think is fueled by fat. Consequently, you start burning your undesirable fat deposits with minimal (dare I say, no?) conscious effort.

WHY IS FAT BURNING SO HARD?

In general, it's pretty difficult to get into the "fat burning mode." Lipolysis and fat oxidation are under *tight* hormonal control. If you know anything about hormones, you know they can make you feel powerless. Hormones can be temperamental, controlling, and moody: one day your best friend, the next your worse enemy. With the whole fat burning thing, they're usually your worst enemy. In its typical hormonal state, the body *loves* to use easy-breezy glucose (sugar from carbs) and glycogen (glucose stored in the muscles) for energy. It also *loves* to preserve stored fat at all costs. Why does the body want to save fat? It goes back to the history of being human.

Today, many of us are fortunate enough to be assured of our next meal. I'm guessing that even if you're stressing about rent and bills like I am, you probably aren't worried about *literally* starving. But while our conscious mind may know food is coming, our physical body does not. For all it knows, you might not eat again for a month! For your body, your limited carb stores signify immediate and easily accessible energy from the food just eaten. Stored fat is "saved" for long-term energy during starvation. (And of course, our highly palatable, high calorie, addictive, and processed diets encourage the body to save these extra calories as fat left and right, which doesn't help matters much.) As noted in *Science* magazine (1999):

> It has been argued that efficient [fat storage] is beneficial because it allows longer survival during famine. However, for many Western populations, where food supply is abundant and readily available, efficient energy storage predisposes to obesity, the accumulation of excess body fat. Obesity affects more than one-third of the U.S. population and is a major public health concern because it is associated with diabetes, hypertension, hyperlipidemia, and cardiovascular disease.

It's like glucose is your "checking account," and fat is your "savings account." Why tap into your savings (fat) if you've got money (glucose and glycogen) in your checking account? Or it's like having a cell phone that you recharge every day (its glucose stores), along with a backup battery on the side (its fat stores). Why use the backup battery as long as the phone itself (glucose stores) still has juice in it?

Indeed, the body does not like tapping into its *precious* fat stores unless it registers starvation, or will need steady energy for a longer amount of time than glucose stores will support, such as on a long walk. If you could just be like, *"Hey body! It's ok! You can burn the fat, and I'll still eat in a few hours!"* then everything would be so much easier. But alas, it does not work that way. So how do we get the benefits of fat burning from "starvation" without actually starving? Welcome intermittent fasting!

ENTERING FAT BURNING MODE

With all the laments of burning fat, your body will *actually start the whole process on its own,* no questions asked! All you have to do is create the proper setting! You see, once the body has gone a good chunk of hours without food from external sources (like a meal or snack), it switches from using stored glucose (sugar) as the primary source of fuel, to fat instead. This starts occurring around 12 hours after your last meal, with fat burning continuing to escalate until 72 hours (at which point it plateaus). This means if you just *wait it out*, your body *will* give in. The crying baby *will* eventually stop crying. When you hit the fasted stated, gone is the confusion of *"am I burning fat, or just my last meal?"* You're burning fat, trust me.

And not only are you burning fat when fasting: you're *really* burning fat. Fasting encourages cells and mechanisms all throughout the body to begin using more fat, rather than glucose, as fuel. This includes muscles, the central nervous system, and the brain! (The body can generate the minimal amount of glucose required for the brain from fat and protein substrates, while supplementing energy requirements with ketones.)

If you're thinking, *"Yeah that's great and all, but who wants to feel like they're starving in order to burn fat? #notworthit,"* have no fear! When you hit the fasted, fat burning state, appetite disappears. Your body gives in, and doesn't even hold a grudge! In fact, it wholeheartedly embraces the fat burning idea! See Chapter 16: *Why Intermittent Fasting Is Easy* for more on that.

STUBBORN FAT

It gets better. You know those especially stubborn fat stores that just won't go away *no matter what you do?* Maybe you're wondering if it's all in your head? Well, it's not. "Stubborn fat" is a real thing. And intermittent fasting can deal with that too. Let's look at the sciency stuff behind stubborn fat, shall we?

Fat stores are "guarded" by many different receptors. These receptors are like locks, while various hormones and neurotransmitters called *catecholamines* (like epinephrine and norepinephrine) serve as keys. The important "locks" for fat burning are alpha-2 and beta-2 receptors. *Alpha-2 receptors* are like locked doors and are quite difficult to open: they discourage fat burning. *Beta-2 receptors* are like open doors with a welcome sign: they encourage fat burning. So for fat loss, remember alpha = bad, beta = good. Stubborn fat has a lot of alpha-2 receptors, and not many beta-2 receptors. On the other hand, normal or "easy" fat stores have a lot of beta-2 receptors, and not many alpha-receptors. Women tend to have lots of alpha receptors on their hips, butt, and thighs, whereas men have more around their abs and midsection.

How does intermittent fasting unlock those tricky alpha receptors? Since I realize this whole business sounds rather complicated and sciency in a not fun way, let's play an imagination game! Let's pretend your body is a building under tight security, with many guards, hallways, doors, and rooms. The rooms are cells, containing fat inside. The rooms with "alpha doors" are locked and hard to open. The rooms with "beta doors" are much easier to open. Catecholamines are the keys to open the doors. The guards in front of the halls are insulin. Now put your imagination cap on!

Rooms = Cells (With Fat Inside!)
Alpha Doors= Hard To Open
Beta Doors = Easy To Open
Keys = Catecholamines
Guards = Insulin

1. Fasting Stops Insulin (The Guard)

For starters, when insulin is present, basically all fat stores are off limits. Fasting lowers insulin, getting rid of the "guard" and encouraging a fat burning state. With insulin gone, you've actually got a chance at unlocking all those doors (the cells containing fat).

2. Fasting Gives You Catecholamines (Keys)

Fasting ramps up catecholamines in the system, so you've got more keys to open those pesky locks. Fasting increases levels of epinephrine (aka: adrenaline), which inhibits alpha-2 receptors, meaning you can actually open those stubborn doors! Epinephrine also increases the metabolic rate in general, letting you grab more fat from the cells, which doesn't hurt.

3. Fasting Increases Blood Flow

At the same time, fasting stimulates blood flow, which is necessary for these catecholamines to actually reach the receptors. (I guess in our strange analogy, you can't just walk through the hallway up to the doors: you've got to coast on a sea of blood?) Fun fact: this is why if you touch places on your body with little fat, it will probably feel warm (from the blood), while pinching a stubborn fat area (like maybe on your waist or hips) likely feels colder. This is also why "fat burning" ab belts *may* actually help you burn more ab fat, by stimulating more blood flow to the area. Now that you know this, you might begin doing the "fat pinch test" like I would do. (*Cold fat! Stubborn! Curses!*)

4. Fasting Increases Fat Burning In General

Of course, opening the doors is one thing. *Burning* the fat inside is another. People who constantly eat carb-rich diets may reach the "fat burning state" with exercise, yet don't necessarily burn that much fat. When the body is accustomed to running on glucose, it "hits the wall" once glycogen storages are almost empty. Even though this is *prime* fat burning time, *you just can't do it* (or so it seems). It's like you *finally* open the doors, and then they catch you on the security cameras and shut down your whole fat burning plan. Alas. But with fasting, the body has "accepted" fat burning, so there's no struggle in actually grabbing and burning the fat. No one's stopping you! You've got the green light!

To summarize our lovely imagination game, intermittent fasting gives you the keys to open stubborn fat cells, and then encourages your body to *actually* burn the fat inside of them.

Intermittent fasting for the win!

But wait, it gets even better….

FAT GAIN PROTECTION

Not only does intermittent fasting yield effortless fat burning, it also makes you less likely to store fat via *enhanced nutrition partitioning*. This means you're more likely to use food for fuel and repair, rather than simply shuttling it away into fat storage.

A 2012 *Cell Metabolism* study on mice obesity compared two groups of mice: one which ate a high fat diet ad libitum throughout the day, and another which ate a high fat diet ad libitum but in a restricted time window, à la intermittent fasting. Even when the two groups consumed *the same amount of calories from the same nutrient sources*, the fasted mice didn't gain excessive weight, unlike the non-fasted mice, who did. Intermittent fasting improved their nutrient utilization by changing catabolic and anabolic pathways and liver metabolism to encourage weight homeostasis, rather than fat storage. The study concluded these "remarkable" findings suggest that time-restricted eating actually "reprograms the molecular mechanisms of energy metabolism and body weight regulation." So much for a calorie is just a calorie!

Another study analyzing the effects of fasting on healthy, normal weight men, found that prolonged fasting increased fat oxidation once the men ate a normal meal again. This means intermittent fasting may cause you to burn more fat when you eat than you would if you ate constantly throughout the day!

FAT BURNING IN MEN VS. WOMEN

While intermittent fasting is stellar for promoting fat burning and discouraging fat storage, there is notably a *marked* difference between how men and women store and use fat, resulting in typically different body shapes. It all goes back to one simple concept: babies.

Ya see, females have to maintain a substantial amount of nutritional energy stores just in case they need to, *oh I don't know*, support another living being inside their body for 9 months? Yep. Females actually favor a higher body fat percentage than males in order to protect the future kids. (The female body just assumes this will happen at some point - good luck convincing it otherwise.) This does insinuate one nifty thing about fat: *it sustains life*! Fat for the win! Try "growing" an infant on processed sugar and see how that goes!

But I digress. Let's explore the many differences in male and female fat metabolism, which just may bring you peace about some of your more stubborn fatty deposits! For starters, women typically have a higher body fat percentage than men. It relates to the whole pregnancy issue discussed above. Women store excess fat in order to support a presumed future baby. Fat = baby food. The fact that women store more fat in the *gluteal-femoral region* (butt and thighs) while men store more fat in the *visceral depot* (midsection and abs) relates to this baby thing. In fact, women easily gain lower body fat but struggle to burn it, because their thigh fat is specifically saved for pregnancy to nurture the infant. This explains why thigh fat can be extremely hard to burn for women, and perhaps why popular culture focuses more on burning ab fat, which is much more "burnable" hormonally. Ladies, this also means you'll more easily lose thigh fat when pregnant! Doing some nice walking while having a bun in the oven just may leave you with leaner legs when all's said and done! (It's actually harder for normal weight men to burn lower body fat as well - it's just *even harder* for women.)

Interestingly yet appropriately, the game changes for women after menopause, when the whole "pregnancy" idea isn't so plausible anymore. Post-menopause, women begin storing more abdominal fat like men. Obesity also levels the playing field, as obese men and women do not feature as many regional differences in fat storage. It seems that fat stored unhealthily in excess gains license to go everywhere. On the flip side, lean men and women with similar amounts of fat around their abs and lower body will release similar amounts of fat from such areas.

After eating, women are more likely to store fat in *subcutaneous tissue*, while men are more likely to store it in *visceral tissue*. Subcutaneous fat is the fat beneath your skin - the stuff you can actually pinch. Visceral fat is the fat deep in your body around your organs, and is more hazardous to your health. This means fat storage after a meal is, in a way, "healthier" for women than men. (Although men release upper subcutaneous fat more easily than women.)

As for fasting and exercise, women experience higher rates of lipolysis while fasting than men, meaning they "free up" more stored fat for fuel. However, women also store more fat after eating, so it's kind of a moot point. Similarly, women burn more energy from fat while exercising than men, who use more glucose. Women also store more fat in their muscles, which is good for sparing glucose in fat-fueled exercise. During exercise, sympathetic activity (epinephrine and norepinephrine) is also higher in women than in men. So women are more "alert," as it were, during exercise.

SO WHAT DOES IT ALL MEAN?

To summarize the *whole-fat-burning-battle-of-the-sexes* thing, yes, women are "fatter" than men, but that fat has a very specific purpose involving the continuation of the species. Women also tend to store excess fat in a "healthy" manner – subcutaneously and around the thighs. Men, on the other hand, tend to store excess fat unhealthily as visceral fat around the abdomen. Women also use fat more easily in times of "good stress" like exercise and fasting. The takeaway is that "fat" is highly context specific, and a bit of "excess" may actually signal good health. (The "pear" shape tends to be healthy, while the "apple" shape… not so much). At the very least, if you're a girl, accept the fact that your thigh fat has a very noble purpose!

CHAPTER NINETEEN

EXERCISE, IF STYLE

So what happens if you add exercise to the whole intermittent fasting and fat burning scenario? While people quickly assume exercising on an empty stomach will hinder performance and encourage exhaustion, studies consistently show quite the opposite.

INCREASED ENDURANCE

When I think of my pre-fasting days, I think of daytime lethargy where an hour long workout equated to *eons*. Perhaps the biggest difference in my life from intermittent fasting is that the idea of "running out of energy" just really isn't a thing anymore. I simply *know* I can keep going, no questions asked. When fasting, you simply don't tire as easily. The whole "nap" concept becomes a distant memory.

There's a reason for this magical endurance. "Typical" non-fasted exercise is fueled by glucose (sugar from carbohydrates) and glycogen (carbohydrates stored in the muscles and liver). The use of glucose and glycogen for fuel during exercise *inhibits fatty acid oxidation*. This not only blunts fat burning in general, but also puts a proverbial ceiling on endurance, since glycogen stores are *quite* limited compared to fat. You can deplete glycogen stores in an intense exercise session, while the average person has enough stored body fat to walk over 1,000 miles! No big deal.

When your body is accustomed to relying primarily on carbohydrates from your relatively-recent last meal, you "hit the wall" when you exhaust that stored glycogen. In fact, you probably will "hit the wall" even *before* complete glycogen depletion, as the brain anticipates running out of glycogen, and slows down physical activity in preparation. (You get tired before you even "run out" of actual energy. Sneaky brain!) In fact, studies suggest that simply *thinking* you're going to "hit the wall" may make you "hit the wall." As Benjamin Rapoport notes in the 2010 *PLoS Computational Biology*, "An apparent paradox of long-distance running is that even the leanest athletes store enough fat to power back-to-back marathons, yet small carbohydrate reservoirs can nevertheless catastrophically limit performance in endurance exercise."

But with fasted exercise, there is no wall! Fasted training upregulates the body's ability to burn fat for fuel, resulting in much more sustainable exercise: the longer you go, the more energy you free up to use! One trial found that rats fasted for 24 hours could run longer than rats in the fed state. Interestingly, the fasted rats could run longer even when blood sugar dropped *below* that of the fed rats: their proverbial "wall" was gone! While the carb-fueled rats "ran out of energy" when they started running out of carbs, the fasted rats easily carried on! The study concluded that fasting increases the use of fats as fuel during exercise, while the corresponding "glycogen sparing" effect increases endurance.

FAT ADAPTATION AND PRESERVED GLUCOSE

As discussed above, studies consistently support the body's preference for fat as fuel during fasted training. A 6 week diet-controlled study in the 1985 *Journal of Applied Physiology*, comparing fasted versus fed exercise, found fasted exercise instigates metabolic adjustments within muscles for fat adaptation. Fasted exercise encourages the muscles to utilize intramyocellular lipids (fat stored in the muscle) for energy, and increases the oxidative capacity of muscle. In other words, fasted training encourages your muscles to use more fat, rather than carbs, as fuel. This prevents the drops in blood sugar which happen during carbohydrate-fueled exercise, when the muscles use more glucose. The study concluded that "regular fasted training is a useful strategy to stimulate physiological adaptations in muscle that may eventually contribute to improve endurance exercise performance."

Another study (1998 *Journal of Applied Physiology*) comparing an overnight fast to a longer 3.5 day fast prior to exercise found fasted training substantially maintained glucose levels. In the longer fast, the body generated more glucose during the first hour of exercise, while ultimately sparing it, relying more on fatty acids and ketones. Insulin levels also lowered, and performance was maintained. As previously discussed, the study found that fasted exercise supports steady blood sugar levels by sparing glucose, encouraging the body to instead rely on fat.

INHIBITED WEIGHT GAIN

Not only does fasted training utilize more fat for energy, it also may protect against weight gain in a *hyper-caloric* state, which is pretty nifty. One study in the 2010 *Journal of Physiology* looked at healthy males eating 30% more calories than needed per day (half of those from fat) for 6 weeks. Some of the men did carb-fueled aerobic training, some did fasted aerobic training, and some didn't train at all. The ones who didn't train gained an average of 3 lbs after 6 weeks, while the ones who trained with carbs gained around 1.5 lbs in 6 weeks. But the men who exercised while fasting, even though they ate more calories than they "burned," gained no weight after 6 weeks! Furthermore, only fasted training increased glucose tolerance and insulin sensitivity. The study concluded that "fasted training is more potent than fed training to facilitate adaptations in muscle and to improve whole-body glucose tolerance and insulin sensitivity during hyper-caloric fat-rich diet."

MUSCLE PRESERVATION

But what about muscle you say? Will fasted training make your muscles waste away? Hardly. Think about the nature of resistance training for a second: straining and breaking the muscle forces it to adapt, and ultimately rebuild itself stronger. Stressing the muscle ultimately *benefits* it. Intermittent fasting is similar in that it stresses the body, and instigates beneficial adaptations.

A 2011 University of Illinois review of 18 studies involving calorie restriction, intermittent fasting, and body composition, found that intermittent fasting patterns favor muscle preservation. While dieting alone averages 25% weight loss from muscle, dieting in intermittent fasting patterns averages only around 10% weight loss from muscle. The study noted that "intermittent restriction regimens may be superior to daily restriction regimens in that they help conserve lean mass at the expense of fat mass."

But that's intermittent fasting coupled with a calorie deficit, and *without* exercise. Since both fasting and exercise individually support favorable gene regulation in regards to muscle adaptations, what happens when you combine the two? The aforementioned review concluded by considering the potential benefits of this idea: "As endurance exercise has been shown to... aid in the retention of lean mass, the combination effects of these two interventions on body weight [intermittent fasting and exercise] and body composition could be a fruitful area for future study."

Studies do indeed support the notion that fasted exercise may support muscle growth. The previously mentioned fasted versus carb-fueled training in a hyper-caloric diet study, found fasted training increased muscle protein content by 28%. Furthermore, a 2010 randomized, crossover study analyzed muscle protein uptake in young males after either fed training (a carb breakfast) or fasted training (an empty stomach). It found that fasted training significantly increased P70S6 kinase, a gene which signals muscle growth. The study concluded that fasted training "may stimulate the intramyocellular anabolic response to ingestion of a carbohydrate/protein/leucine mixture following a heavy resistance training session." In other words, fasted training may actually prime your muscles for growth! On top of all that, remember that fasting promotes *autophagy*, or the recycling of old and damaged proteins within the body for new growth and repair. Autophagy is actually required to maintain muscle mass. Oh hey!

With all that said, if you're *still* worried about your muscles while fasting, you can always supplement with BCAAs (amino acids) during the fasting period as a sort of "insurance," à la Martin Berkhan's *Leangains* protocol.

SO WHAT DOES IT ALL MEAN?

To recap, exercising while fasted ramps up fat burning and provides an abundance of energy, especially when compared to finicky and controlling carbohydrate stores. Muscles become more adept at using fat as fuel, and glucose is spared. Endurance and stamina increase. Protein is preserved, protecting and supporting existing muscle.

Think of it like *Titanic*. (Go with me on this: I seriously mused on it for an unnaturally long time.)

Rose = The Body
Leo = Fat Stores
Cal (Rose's Rich Fiancé) = Carb Stores

Who sticks around? Who's always there? Sure, Cal AKA Carbs may give Rose pretty things and provide an occasional motivational boost, but in the end, he shuns and forsakes her. He's even like, *"Hey, I'll help out Leo AKA Fat"*... but it's all lies. It's akin to that false boost of energy from sugar, which convinces you that you'll finally burn fat because *you're just so energetic for ever and ever!* Then you crash and burn. Fail. Sneaky carbs. And where is Cal AKA Carbs when things get real and the ship is sinking? Yeah that's right. He's not there. But guess who's *always* there for you! That's right! Leo AKA Fat! Even when you can't actually see him! (Like when you haven't eaten in awhile, or, in the case of Leo, he's dead.)

Pick who you want. I'm going with Leo AKA Fat on this one.

CHAPTER TWENTY

INTERMITTENT FASTING Q&A

Got Intermittent Fasting questions? I've got answers! For unaddressed thoughts, feel free to contact me via *WhatWhenWine.com*.

IF PROTOCOL QUESTIONS

What Is Intermittent Fasting?
Intermittent fasting is a dietary protocol in which you restrict the hours you eat, rather than the amount of food you eat. Most people end up eating in a time period of around 6-10 hours each day.

How Long Should I/Can I Fast?
The possibilities really are endless. Fat burning and its benefits begin after 12 hours or so. (A 12 hour fast is therefore recommended at minimum.) Between 16 and 24 hours is a sort of "golden time" in which fat burning continues to rapidly escalate, and in which you typically feel more alert and energetic the longer you go. Fat burning continues to rise until 72 hours, at which point most metabolic

adaptations have been fully realized, and fatty acid release plateaus. (This is just for information purposes. With intermittent fasting, you rarely go longer than 24 hours.) The more weight you have to lose, the longer you can probably go with ease. Pick a protocol and go with it, knowing you can always fast longer if you want! Do what feels right.

Is Intermittent Fasting The Same As Longer Fasts?

No. With intermittent fasting, you still eat each day. A 3 day water fast, for example, is *not* "intermittent fasting" as referred to by the IF community. That is an actual fast. Nor is a juice fast the same as intermittent fasting. That's just restricting the *type* of food you eat, rather than the *time* you eat.

How Much Do I Eat In The Eating Window?

During the eating window, you can eat all you want! Don't stress about "eating enough" or "getting enough calories." Simply eat to satiety, and you'll be fine. If you do actually need to eat more, you'll be more hungry the next time you eat. Your body is smart like that.

How Much Water Should I Drink While Fasting?

Don't stress about water. Drink so that you're not thirsty. I always have a water bottle with me, and sip on it as needed. Use your urine color as a gauge. If it's nice, light, and clear like pale lemonade, then you're good. If it's super yellow like gatorade, then you probably should drink more water.

Can I Eat Anything During The Fasting Period?

Unfortunately, no. Doing so breaks the fast. Having "just a little bite" to ward off hunger will only lengthen the transition into fat burning, and actually increase appetite in the long run. Don't do it. It really doesn't help, I promise!

Can I Drink Coffee Or Tea During The Fast?

Yes you can! Doing so may even ease the transition into fasting. I practically lived on tea and coffee my first week or so of intermittent fasting. Ideally you shouldn't add any milk or cream, but if you simply *must*, then cap it at a tablespoon or so. As long as its a fairly negligible amount, it probably won't hinder your fast. (Plus the caffeine in the drink will rev up your metabolism, encouraging fat burning.) Only use zero calorie sweeteners. Do NOT put sugar in your drink. (I personally found that once I cut out sweetened coffee and tea, fasting actually became even easier. Now I simply take green tea or caffeine pills in the morning.)

Can I Have Other Non-Caloric Drinks During The Fast?

If you're just doing IF and not Paleo, then zero calorie drinks like diet sodas (*Oh hey my former lover, Coke Zero!*) and sugar-free water enhancers *are* acceptable during the fast. If you're combining IF with Paleo like I do, you'll want to avoid processed drinks and just stick with water, coffee, tea, or something like lemonade made from water, lemon juice, and stevia.

What Other Supplements Help With Fasting?

I encourage supplements which increase your metabolism and upregulate fat burning, rather than merely masking appetite. Caffeine, L-tyrosine, ginseng, Rhodiola, and Gingko biloba are all good for this. See Chapter 24: *Supplements* for details.

What Else Helps With Fasting?

Physical activity and staying busy help fasting (especially in the beginning stages) by "distracting" you, while also encouraging fat for fuel use. Check out Chapter 14: *Tips For Intermittent Fasting* for more.

How Should I Break The Fast?

Some say to "lightly" break the fast with vegetables or fruit. I personally break the fast with whatever I'm feeling at the moment, be it meat, vegetables, or perhaps a glass of wine. You'll find what works best for you, especially since fasting makes you more "in tune" with your body. And since fasting primes the body for enhanced nutrition partitioning, whatever you *do* eat in your feeding window will more likely be used for fuel and repair, rather than immediate fat storage. Fasting functions like insurance, in a way!

What About Eating Out?

You may think intermittent fasting will dampen your social life, but it doesn't have to! Most people settle on protocols which include lunch and/or dinner. If you're doing a night-eating protocol like me, then dinners with friends are not only an option, but now *guilt free!* It's quite fun to confidently order and enjoy the massive steak, to the surprise of onlookers, especially on dates! (Guys always think I'll order the salad, and then are in awe of my carnivorous nature.

Although I've never dated a Vegan, which I suppose could be slightly problematic.)

For the times that the fasting window does unavoidably conflict with a social function, you can always choose for yourself when to take days off. I'm in such an ingrained pattern, that I often suggest coffee or tea in place of breakfast or lunch, making allowances for special occasions like holiday brunches. In any case, intermittent fasting is just that: *intermittent*. You can change it up and do different meals here and there to your pleasing! IF should be ultimately freeing, not restricting!

IF FEARS QUESTIONS

Will I Die?

No. At least not from intermittent fasting. If you do, it *wasn't* intermittent. You would die from fasting after completely depleting your fat stores. We're talking at minimum, a month of eating *nothing* if you were already super lean, and possibly up to a year if you were obese.

Won't Fasting Make Me Lethargic?

Nope. You'll actually be alert and energetic! Fasting saturates the body with energy by ramping up lipolysis, which is the breakdown of stored fats into potential energy. It literally shifts the body into an energy-producing mode! The longer you fast, the more fatty acids are produced. Fasting can even release up to 200-300% *more* fatty acids into the bloodstream from fat stores than needed! (The ultimately unused fatty acids are simply restored or used elsewhere in the body.

Won't I Be Miserably Hungry When Fasting?

Nope. You actually will likely have *zero* appetite when fasting. Zilch. You know that feeling when you lose your appetite because you're excited about something, or in love/like/lust? It's kind of like that. Fasting boosts levels of adrenaline, while limitless fuel comes from body fat stores and ketones. You won't be hungry when fasting because you'll be filled with fuel from within! (Not in a vague esoteric sense, but rather in an actual sense.) Your body even "tells" you it doesn't need to eat by killing appetite!

Won't My Metabolism Slow Down? What About "Starvation Mode?"

Oh, how haunted are we by the dreadful "starvation mode!" We MUST eat a certain amount of calories consistently, otherwise our body will assume we're starving, our metabolism will slow down, and we won't lose ANY weight.

Don't worry - it's all lies. The metabolism "slows down" in response to calorie restriction, not time restriction. If you undergo calorie restriction for a substantial period of time (which is not the basic form of intermittent fasting), the metabolic rate will lower to compensate. It will not, however, "shut off" completely or enter some irrevocable mode where fat burning ceases all together. Fat loss will simply just occur at a slower rate. Even then, it's not a permanent nor even problematic situation.

And that's just calorie restriction! As for intermittent fasting, since the metabolic rate does *not* decrease in response to time intervals between meals as long as adequate nutrients are consumed for the day, you will *not* enter some nefarious "starvation mode" when fasting. In fact, some studies even show that short-term fasting increases metabolic rate (go figure). Skipping a meal will surely not slow your metabolism, nor will going 24 hours without a meal! I do it all the time, and my metabolism is just dandy! For a more thorough explanation, see Chapter 17: *The Myths of Metabolism*.

Will I Lose Muscle From Fasting?

Fasting actually spares lean muscle tissue by mobilizing fat and ketones as alternative substrates to protein. As noted in the 2012 *American Journal of Physiology - Endocrinology and Metabolism*, regarding fasting: "Lipolysis, lipid oxidation, ketone body synthesis, tailored endogenous glucose production and uptake, and decreased glucose oxidation serve to protect against excessive erosion of protein mass." Furthermore, fasting promotes autophagy, which is actually required to maintain muscle mass. If you still feel paranoid, you can always supplement with amino acids during the fast.

Will I Overeat In My Feeding Window?

The short answer is: highly unlikely. The slightly longer answer is: highly unlikely, but even if you did, it probably wouldn't matter that much anyway. Studies find that fasting decreases appetite and does *not* instigate compensatory overeating. On the contrary, people are actually more likely to *undereat* in total when practicing intermittent fasting (which in the grand scheme of things, is more of a good thing than a bad thing). Even if you do "overeat" per se, fasting encourages enhanced nutrient partitioning, so food is more likely to be used for fuel and repair rather than fat storage. Studies show that mice who overeat after fasting do not gain weight like mice who overeat in a non-fasted pattern. And if you couple intermittent fasting with the extremely satiating Paleo diet, overconsumption of food during your "feasting" is *extremely* unlikely.

Will I Automatically Store Everything As Fat After Fasting?
Quite the opposite. After a fast has ended, the body experiences increased nutrient partitioning, and is less likely to store food as fat, even in excess. When fat storage does occur after fasting, it is also more likely to happen in other areas besides fat cells, such as muscles, where it can then be used as energy. Studies also show that eating after a fast increases total fat oxidation from the meal in comparison to eating in a "normal" meal pattern.

Won't Intermittent Fasting Be HARD?
Nope. Intermittent Fasting is almost laughably easy. See Chapter 16: *Why Intermittent Fasting Is Easy* for more on that!

What Type Of Intermittent Fasting Do You Do?
I do a dinner only protocol. I begin eating at dinner, whenever that happens to be for that particular day, and then munch afterwards until bed. I love it! I go to bed full, yet wake up raring to go in the fasted state! Talk about easy breezy!

Part Three

Wine?

CHAPTER TWENTY-ONE

ALCOHOL AND DIET

Most diet plans forbid alcohol. Even standard Paleo discourages it (oops). I am of the opinion, however, that one must live life to the fullest, adopting a diet protocol sustainably enjoyable. Is there a way to have your drink and drink it too? Yes! I regularly consume alcohol in the form of red wine, a habit I actually developed *after* going Paleo. I am also at my thinnest and healthiest. Studies consistently link moderate alcohol consumption to longevity and healthy biomarkers, even more so than teetotalers!

ALCOHOL BENEFITS

There are a myriad of benefits associated with alcohol consumption. For starters, moderate alcohol consumption is linked to increased lifespan. It improves insulin sensitivity and discourages insulin resistance, particularly in women. It protects the heart from cardiovascular disease and is preventative against metabolic syndrome (again, particularly in women), positively affecting blood lipids and waist circumference. It may be preventative against rheumatoid arthritis and neurological diseases such as Alzheimer's and stroke. Mentally, moderate alcohol consumption can positively affect stress and depression. As for my personal favorite, alcohol has been shown to be protective against the common cold! Oh hey!

ALCOHOL FAT BURNING AND STORAGE

Alcohol has *quite* a paradoxical relationship with body weight. A macronutrient high in calories, alcohol contains 7.1 calories per gram, ranking it near fat's 9 calories per gram. On the one hand, studies show that drinking alcohol with a meal does *not* instigate a compensatory decrease in food calories. In other words, if you have a drink with dinner, you probably won't eat less to "make up for it." Alcohol also minimizes fat oxidation when consumed. Such factors would seem to correlate alcohol with weight gain.

But that's just not the case.

Calories from alcohol do not act like "normal" calories. Studies show that substituting calories from carbohydrates with calories from alcohol typically leads to *weight loss*, while calories consumed in excess from alcohol don't necessarily result in weight gain. (So much for the "calorie is just a calorie" theory.) In fact, hospitalized alcoholics gained NO weight when *1800 calories* in the form of alcohol was added to their standard diet. A similar metabolic ward study found that substituting 50% of the patients' daily calories with alcohol yielded weight loss. Furthermore, while adding 2,000 calories of chocolate to a patient's diet steadily increased weight (shocker), adding 2,000 calories of alcohol *negligibly* affected weight. Such results indicate alcohol may exhibit protective mechanisms against weight gain.

The reasons for alcohol's paradoxical effects on weight are widely debated. Theories range from alcohol's thermogenic effect (which is around 20%), an increase in metabolism (adding alcohol can increase the basal metabolic rate by around 5%), enhanced ATP breakdown, a "wasting" of the calories from alcohol, or perhaps a long-term reduction in food intake beyond a single meal. Whatever the case, moderate consumption of alcohol may be ultimately protective against obesity, particularly in women.

ALCOHOL METABOLISM

Alcohol is burned preferentially in the body over other fuel substrates (fats, carbs, and protein). It does *not* easily become body fat. No simple or practical pathway exists for alcohol to fatty acid conversion. In the worst case scenario, around 5% of alcohol could *possibly* be converted to fat, although such is unlikely. When you imbibe, it's not the alcohol which actually becomes body fat: it's whatever you consume *with* your drink which shows up on the proverbial scale. (Not that we support scales around here!) Weight gain from drinking stems from sugary, caloric mixers and loss of inhibitions, as healthy diet pledges go out the window. Hello fast food binge, validated via excuses of needing something to "soak up the alcohol!" (I shudder thinking about the many times my college friends and I hit up *Denny's* for pancakes, or *Jack In the Box* for a large bucket of curly fries, circa 3 AM.)

RED WINE

While moderate alcohol consumption boasts a myriad of benefits, red wine in particular increases the healthy effects. Consider "The French Paradox," encompassing the idea that the French diet is high in saturated fat, yet low in heart disease. A prominent theory attributes this "paradox" to the population's moderate consumption of red wine. (Check out Chapter 5: *Fat Problems* for more on the saturated fat/heart disease issue.) A 2009 *Journal of Epidemiology & Community Health* study analyzing different alcoholic drinks and longevity, found that wine in particular most strongly correlated to longer lifespan and decreased heart disease, increasing average life expectancy by 5 years. 70% of the wine consumed in the data was red wine. In fact, studies on dealcoholized red (but not white) wine confirm its cardiovascular benefits.

What makes red wine so special?

In addition to alcohol's health benefits, red wine contains *phenolic acids* and *polyphenols*. The most famous of these is *resveratrol*, a polyphenol found within the grape skin. The amount of resveratrol varies from wine to wine and can be relatively low, a possible explanation for why moderate consumption of wine is more beneficial than light consumption or complete abstinence. Wines produced in the areas of southwestern France and Sardinia yield the highest amounts of resveratrol, where production methods specifically preserve the compound. The population of these areas, geographically, are also associated with increased longevity. (This is all correlational, of course.)

RESVERATROL

Let's take a look at the many potential benefits of wine's most famous and potent polyphenol, christened "resveratrol."

1. Resveratrol And Heart Health

While moderate consumption of red wine in general reduces the risk of coronary heart disease, resveratrol is specifically cardio-protective. Animals given dealcoholized red wine exhibited the same cardiac benefits as those administered pure resveratrol, suggesting such polyphenols found in wine exert their own cardio-protective properties separate from those of alcohol.

Resveratrol protects the heart by minimizing oxidative stress, hypertension, heart failure, cardiomyopathy, atherosclerosis, diabetes, obesity, and other cardiac dysfunctions. It supports heart health by encouraging autophagy in heart-related processes, and activation of an anti-inflammatory protein in the heart called Sirtuin 1.

2. Resveratrol And Anti-Aging

Like calorie restriction, resveratrol is heralded for its anti-aging effects, altering metabolic pathways to improve insulin sensitivity. It also activates multiple longevity genes (with fancy names like SIRT and FOX01), prevents age-related cardiovascular decline, and extends lifespan in general.

3. Resveratrol Acts Like Exercise

This one may be my favorite! While a glass of red wine won't build muscle or burn pre-existing fat stores, it may act like exercise in the body! In a 2011 study published in *The FASEB Journal*, scientists were trying to find a way to prevent atrophy, bone mineral density loss, and other negative effects arising from an astronaut's lack of weight-bearing exercise in zero gravity. The scientists found that resveratrol "prevents the wasting disorders of mechanical unloading by acting as a physical exercise mimetic in the rat." In other words, resveratrol seems to have an exercise-like effect in the body! The scientists simulated the sedentary effects of the weightless lifestyle by hanging rats by their hind legs (poor things). While the hanging control rats experienced loss of muscle and increased insulin resistance from their lack of movement, the rats fed resveratrol were fully protected from such. The study concluded that resveratrol may counteract the negative effects of a sedentary lifestyle by acting as an exercise mimetic.

Furthermore, a 2012 study in the *Journal of Physiology* found that resveratrol supplementation enhanced the beneficial effects of exercise, and increased endurance rates in rats. As the study notes, "Resveratrol, an antioxidant found in red wine, has beneficial effects on cardiac and skeletal muscle function, similar to the effects of endurance exercise training." So having a glass of red wine *may* just make up for not hitting the gym! (Although my thoughts on the gym are slightly complicated anyways. See Chapter 22: *"Functional" Exercise* for more on that.)

4. Other Resveratrol Benefits
Like a "miracle compound," resveratrol also boasts estrogenic, antiplatelet, antioxident, and anti-inflammatory properties, inhibiting COX1 and COX2 gene expression. These anti-inflammatory properties may counteract osteoarthritis and protect cells from degenerative diseases. In fact, resveratrol may be especially protective against cancer, inhibiting cancerous cells at all stages: initiation, promotion, and progression.

OTHER POLYPHENOLS

And resveratrol isn't the only polyphenol found in red wine. There are over 200 documented phenolic compounds, although further research is needed for the various potential benefits of such. One compound called *piceatannol*, for example, may help with weight loss. Piceatannol actually discourages the formation of new fat cells by shutting off pathways needed for immature fat cells to grow. While baby fat cells can take 10 days to mature, their growth is stunted (and possibly stopped altogether) by piceatannol. If that's not awesome, I don't know what is!

THE PALEO ALCOHOL CLUB?

You may believe that joining the Paleo club will demand alcohol abstinence, and that you'll be sadly screaming *"You can't sit with us!"*

Mean Girls style to any stiff drink who approaches the table. While it's true that not all Paleo protocols support our spirited friend, my version of Paleo definitely fancies some variety in the drink department! As discussed above, I support red wine as the ultimate alcoholic "health" drink, with white wine arriving in second place. If the vino stuff isn't your proverbial cup of tea, choose clear liquors à la gin, vodka, or tequila, imbibed straight-up or with non-offensive mixers like club soda and lime. The *"Norcal Margarita"* is a common drink in Paleoland, consisting of tequila, lime juice/pulp, and club soda to taste.

SO WHAT DOES IT ALL MEAN?

Alcohol is quite the paradox. On the plus side, moderate alcohol intake provides a myriad of health benefits, and is linked to increased longevity overall. Red wine in particular supports heart health, discourages weight gain, and may even act like exercise in a glass! And while quite caloric, alcohol *in and of itself* does not encourage fat gain, nor inhibit weight loss. Weight gain from drinking comes from whatever else is consumed *with* the alcohol. So yes, you *can* have your drink and drink it too… unless you binge on unhealthy foods while drinking. Self control and moderation is key! Use good judgement, and drink on!

PART FOUR
And?

Chapter Twenty-Two

"Functional" Exercise

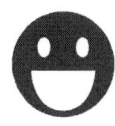

I'm always shocked yet sincerely flattered when people ask me if I do ballet, giving a nod to my "dancer's body." I graciously receive such compliments, which connote adjectives like thin, toned, and graceful. Alas, I am not a dancer. Never having taken dance classes is actually one of my very few regrets in life thus far. Similarly, people will inquire about my workout routine and which gym I attend, since I'm in "such good shape." The thing is, I don't really have one. Not anymore. Not since realizing that the foundation of body composition stems from "diet" rather than "exercise," and that consistent *movement* can be more efficacious than concentrated bouts of cardio.

Believe it or not, suffering at the gym is not necessarily necessary to reap and maintain a thin, toned body. Diet and lifestyle ultimately determine the body's preference for fat burning and storage, protein and muscle synthesis, and use of "calories" in general. Ergo, careful food choices can establish a hormonal profile on a cellular level which favors a beautiful composition. Even with hundreds of crunches, muscles will remain buried treasures if lying beneath a layer of white adipose tissue. And even with hours of cardio, this white adipose tissue may linger if one eats foods in a pattern encouraging fat storage.

These days, I rarely do crunches or cardio, yet maintain a toned physique. I simply focus on dietary choices (Paleo) and patterns (intermittent fasting) which encourage fat burning, while sprinkling in bits of "functional exercise," as I shall discuss. (Hint: It involves exercising without "exercising," per se.)

Note: In this chapter I'm using "exercise" to mean going to a gym, performing a set workout for a "certain" amount of time in order to burn a "certain" amount of calories, and then going home. I do not mean actively moving around the world as a part of *life*, which I wholeheartedly support!

THE MYTH OF CARDIO

Before I got my diet in line, I'd work out in the gym, cardio junkie style, *a lot*. While these sweaty efforts never seemed to make a substantial dent in my body composition or touch those love handles, I just figured I "wasn't doing enough." After all, the cardio concept makes perfect sense in theory: burn a certain amount of calories, and burn fat! But it just doesn't pan out that way in real life. Unless you're living a cardio *lifestyle* like marathon runners or similar athletes, simple cardio sessions are not the ideal method to blast the fat. Here's why:

1. Our Bodies Are Remarkable At Homeostasis
Creating a "calorie deficit" by burning more calories via cardio is pretty difficult in real life. Studies constantly show that cardio does *not* result in the anticipated weight loss. In general, the body defends a certain weight (or "energy status") *regardless* of daily fluctuations in calorie intake and energy expenditure. Over 6-10 weeks, a typical person's weight will only fluctuate by 0.5%. That's a VERY small change. Even over longer periods, weight adjustments aren't generally very significant. A 2009 *PLOS ONE* study of sedentary, overweight postmenopausal women found that substantially increasing amounts of exercise yielded only *half* of the predicted weight loss. Furthermore, the "exercisers" lost no more body fat than the "non-exercisers."

Think about *you*, for a second. If you're like most people, you probably "hover" around a certain weight for quite awhile. Do you think you *literally* consumed and burned the same amount of calories at the end of each day to perfectly maintain that weight? Highly unlikely. Your body can easily compensate for fluctuating levels of calories burned via exercise without you even realizing, thus maintaining homeostasis.

2. The Body Often Responds To Cardio By Increasing Hunger And/Or Decreasing Activity

Cardio creates a temporary "energy deficit." While individual responses vary, the body often initiates compensatory measures, like increased appetite or reduced activity for the rest of the day, to "make up for" this perceived loss. As observed in *Medicine & Science in Sports & Exercise*, "Exercise-induced perturbations to energy balance may initiate behavioral compensatory adjustments and either alter food intake or cause a reduction in normal daily activities. This compensation for the exercise-induced energy deficit may explain why exercise alone often does not result in successful weight loss…"

In fact, studies show concentrated bouts of "exercise" can actually *change food perception and desire*, making food literally more palatable in the mind. Such signals encourage overcompensation of food, effectively "voiding" fat burning, at least in the "calories in vs. calories out" game. People also often respond to cardio by lounging around the rest of the day, nullifying earlier movement.

3. If You're Counting Calories, Cardio Just Doesn't Burn That Many Of Them

Even if calories *were* the defining factor, cardio just doesn't burn that many of them. Most people burn a couple hundred calories doing cardio at the gym, which is easily "undone" by a sweetened beverage or a few tablespoons of butter. Heck, even a banana may do it! And if your glycogen stores are full when you commence cardio (likely), you might solely utilize the carbs stored in your muscles, never even touching fat. Sad day.

4. And That Said, Cardio And The Whole Calories Thing is Quite Vague

It's difficult to sufficiently gauge calories in vs. calories out on a given day in order to create a deficit via cardio. Even if you "know" that you burned 300 calories on the treadmill (which you don't), you may subsequently move less than you normally would throughout the rest of the day. Or you may have a day with no conscious cardio, yet simply "fidget" more. A 1986 study conducted by Dr. Eric Ravussin at the National Institutes of Health, for example, found that fidgeting could account for 100-800 calories burned per day!) Basically, the amount of calories you "burn" per day from exercise is quite vague, with its effect on your overall daily metabolic rate even vaguer. Check out my concluding thoughts on "NEAT" below.

5. Diet = Always, Exercise = Sometimes

So simple, yet so significant. Unless you're a pro athlete or body builder, you're *probably* "not exercising" more than you're "exercising." On the contrary, you're *always* doing diet. Always. When you eat: that's part of diet. When you don't eat: that's also part of diet! And it's this diet, not exercise, which most determines your body's hormonal preference for fat storage and "set" weight. As they say, *"You can't out-exercise a bad diet."*

Note: With the above points, I'm trying to express why cardio exercise may be ineffective for weight loss specifically. I'm not saying, "Don't exercise!" or "Don't go to the gym!" And while I don't believe insane cardio is incredibly healthy, it's definitely better than being a couch potato! The takeaway is that cardio for fun and stress management and routine can be fantastic, but cardio to burn off calories for fat loss may be less effective than anticipated.

STILL WANT TO BURN FAT WITH CARDIO?

To sum up the problems with cardio, your body will likely view it as divergent from the norm, and respond with panicky freak-out countermeasures which erase your hard work. One study credited the lack of predicted weight loss from cardio to a "compensatory increase in energy intake in response to a *perceived state of relative energy insufficiency."* In other words, concentrated bouts of cardio "exercise" register as a threat to energy levels, which are "limited" in a body running primarily on sugar (AKA carbs). When you start exercising in this constrained state, your body is just like, *"Umm…no."* It then slows you down psychologically and/or ramps up appetite. You just can't win.

Except you can!

The way around this tricky problem is to convince the body that *there is no energy deficit* in the first place, so it will continue burning fat with no questions asked! This occurs when following a lower carb diet (Paleo) or when fasting (IF). Both methods encourage a fat burning state utilizing dietary *and* body fat, allowing you to reassure your body that it has adequate energy, while sneakily imposing a deficit. If you perform cardio when already in the fat burning mode, your body is like, *"Well, good thing we've got tons of fatty acids to fuel this! Keep them coming!"* That's right, since you are already burning fat, you just keep doing it, but more so! Even better, since you're *not* fueled by limited carbs, you won't be filled with a seemingly insatiable appetite to refill them afterwards! See Chapter 19: *Exercise, IF Style* for more on the subject!

And if cardio is indeed your obsession, I've personally found two tricks to *really* maximize fat burning from such. The first is to engage in some light (or not so light) cardio *near the end of your fast* (preferably after 16 or more hours). At such a time, your body is *rocking* the fat burning mode, so it's incredibly effective for effortless fat burning and tapping into those particularly stubborn fat reserves.

Also consider trying some *"High Intensity Interval Training,"* known in the fitness world as HIIT. This is where you alternate brief periods of running at peak intensity, with brief recovery periods of walking or jogging. HIIT encourages maximum fat burning with minimum time investment. Were this an exercise book, I would elaborate with the science and studies. (Like a 2008 one in *Applied Physiology, Nutrition, and Metabolism,* which concluded HIIT was a "powerful method to increase whole-body and skeletal muscle capacities to oxidize fat and carbohydrate in previously untrained individuals." Perhaps in the future!)

"FUNCTIONAL" EXERCISE

After reading all of the above, it may seem like I'm saying dieting is everything, while movement is nothing. Not at all. *Movement is vital.* The problem arrives when we quarantine movement to a sequestered time frame in the day, like some magical quota to fill. On the contrary, I believe physical movement should be *life*. We should run and lift and play out of the joy of moving through the universe, out of the requirements of daily tasks and purposes. As such, I believe the best exercise comes from *enhancing* our natural movements in life.

"FUNCTIONAL" EXERCISE: CARDIO

These days I never consciously perform "cardio." Instead, I set up my body hormonally to burn fat via Paleo and intermittent fasting, and then focus on *consciously moving* throughout the day. Intermittent fasting radically changes your exercise perspective. Once you realize fat burning can occur without running for hours on a treadmill, cardio becomes substantially less appealing. Set your body up to burn fat throughout the day, and you can make every movement you do a sort of "fat burning exercise." Before I began Paleo and intermittent fasting, I was content with lounging around. Sitting was fun. What better way to pass the time than watch TV? Now, you have to strap me down. I stand rather than sit. I fidget. I remain active. I must move constantly. It's like this weird thing.

"FUNCTIONAL" EXERCISE: STRENGTH TRAINING

Just the other day, a woman approached me to say I had the most toned and amazing arms she had ever seen. She wanted to know what weight lifting protocol I followed. Well here it is! It's a bit crazy and seemingly silly, but it gets the job done effortlessly!

1. Body Weights

This is my "big secret." *I wear body weights in my daily home life.* While typing on the computer, cooking, cleaning, doing laundry, or whatever else I may be doing, I simply strap on 1-2 pound wrist weights and 3-4 pound ankle weights. In this way, daily living becomes a form of strength exercise! It also "works out" the muscles used practically in daily life! How perfect is that?

2. Ab Belt

I don't wear an ab belt to "burn stomach fat," but rather to keep me conscious of my core. This encourages me to maintain good posture and contract my ab muscles.

3. Pick Up Stuff

It may seem frivolous, but I also *pick up things* as much as I can. As my family knows, I *love* carrying stuff. Any chance I get to carry something heavy, I do so. Groceries are my favorite. (Always use a basket instead of a cart!) Essentially, I strive to build and maintain muscle through daily tasks.

A "NEAT" FINAL THOUGHT

To conclude my "life as exercise" thesis, consider a neat little thing called "NEAT." This fitting acronym for "Non-Exercise Activity Thermogenesis" refers to all the movement we do outside of conscious "exercise." It's the organic stuff like fidgeting, contracting muscles, and sitting up straight. As James A. Levine at Mayo Clinic Rochester eloquently says, "NEAT includes all those activities that render us vibrant, unique, and independent beings, such as going to work, playing guitar, toe-tapping, and dancing."

To understand NEAT, you must first understand *metabolism*. Check out Chapter 17: *The Myths of Metabolism* for a thorough discussion of the topic, but essentially, the amount of calories "burned" in total per day includes the *Basal Metabolic Rate* (amount of calories required to support body function at rest), *Thermic Effect of Food* (calories burned through digestion and nutrient processing), and *Physical Activity* for any given day. This last one, physical activity, includes both *Volitional Activity* like sports and exercise, as well as *NEAT*, the thermogenesis from movements which aren't conscious "exercise."

NEAT can account for some pretty substantial calorie burning. Studies estimate that two adults of similar body weight can vary in how much they "burn" in a day by 2,000 calories worth of NEAT. *That's 2,000 potential calories you didn't even realize you burned!*

A 1999 *Science* trial analyzed the role of NEAT in 16 average weight patients (12 male and 4 female) ages 25-36, who consumed *1,000 extra calories per day for 8 weeks*, without consciously changing their physical activity. On average, half of the extra 1,000 calories resulted in fat storage, while, on average, half were seemingly "burned" through NEAT. Fat gain in the patients over the course of the trial varied. At the lowest end, one patient gained *less than 1 pound* over the 8 weeks of overfeeding. At the highest end, one patient gained *over 9 pounds*. (Both of these fly in the face of the whole "calories in vs calories out" theory, since "technically" all patients should have gained about 16 pounds.)

The difference in calories burned each day was attributed mostly to NEAT, rather than the other aspects of metabolism discussed above. As such, NEAT was the main factor in resistance to weight gain during overfeeding. The study showed an average increase of 336 calories burned from NEAT per day, ranging individually from 98 to 692 calories. As for the guy who burned the most through NEAT each day (692 calories), the study notes this fat-gain protection from NEAT was the equivalent of "strolling" (or such similar activity) for 1/4 of all waking hours. How delightful!

So what determines NEAT? It may be regulated by a central mechanism in the brain which ramps up NEAT during periods of overeating, and suppresses it during periods of underfeeding. It also seems to vary genetically by person. Those with "naturally" good NEAT activation will be less likely to store fat than those with lower levels of NEAT activation.

For me, NEAT confirms that counting calories and cardio is a nebulous path for weight loss. Sure you can try to gauge how much you *think* you ate or burned that day, but in the end, you just have *no way of knowing*. So perhaps it's better to assume a dietary protocol and lifestyle which encourages fat burning, and then just live your magically wondrous, moving life!

TIPS TO ENHANCE NEAT

1. Add a pep to your step, or walk like you're late to an appointment.

2. Take the stairs rather than the escalator.

3. Do things with intensity and purpose.

4. Sit up straight. (Consider wearing an ab or posture belt during the day, so you're aware of contracting your muscles.)

5. Always stand rather than sit when applicable. If you have a desk job, consider investing in a standing desk. (I actually just use a music stand.) If that's not an option, make a point to get up for a few minutes each hour to stretch and get the blood flowing.

6. Fidget.

7. Explore your world.

8. If it fits into your schedule and commute, consider going to the grocery store daily rather than stocking up. Take a few extra steps around the aisles! And carry a basket!

9. Park far away in the parking lot.

10. Wear whatever shoes encourage you to move the most.

11. Go to that party.

12. Kiss the guy or girl.

13. Dance through Disneyland.

14. Embrace your life.

15. Have fun.

CHAPTER TWENTY-THREE

#DEALING WITH DIET BACKLASH

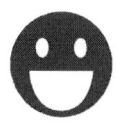

I debated on whether or not to include this chapter, fearing it may come off as #skinnygirlproblems. But as it's an important issue resonating with me, and which I think can help others, here goes!

I used to think in order to be "skinny," you would have to either exist in a state of deleteriously constant hunger, or exercise with an addictive mania. But the more I experimented and tweaked my nutrition, the more I realized that perhaps this wasn't necessarily the case. In researching the *science* of fat usage in the body, I begin to comprehend that "controlling" (for lack of a better word) what you eat, ultimately determines appetite and body composition, not to mention health! Conscious choices to forgo processed foods and sugar, or to regulate eating "windows," can yield a state in which the body receives all needed nutrients while effortlessly burning fat, yielding a slender body satisfied by "basic" foods (by today's standards), and free of cravings.

My new regime rendered me healthy and happy. I *finally* didn't weigh myself or count calories. I ate *all I wanted* when I did eat, with no desire for previously adored (toxic) goodies. I was eating *what* I wanted, *when* I wanted. Rather than looking in the mirror and seeing the weight I wanted to lose, I looked in the mirror and smiled. Yet I occasionally face backlash from family and friends. Accusations of anorexia and "control." Insinuations of disorder and hints of neurosis. Indeed, the trials and tribulations of #skinnygirlproblems can be just as difficult as the backlash for being overweight. While I don't struggle with the actual weight loss anymore, I often struggle with how to approach the topic.

The food choices readily available in today's society easily encourage overeating of fattening foods, leading to the obesity epidemic and majority of today's health problems. Yet society often dismisses overindulging in these sugary, fatty tantalizations as normal, or perhaps even a sign of confidence. Consciously refusing such problematic foods may be viewed as uncanny, unnecessarily restrictive, and unhealthy. While I do believe it's fantastic when people are confident about their bodies, that doesn't make an unhealthy eating lifestyle a *good* thing. Unhealthy eating should not be equated with confidence. The flipside applies as well, and unhealthy restricted eating is just as dangerous. I guess I'm just trying to say it's about health here, not a certain weight.

#DIETBACKLASH

At the beginning of a diet lifestyle change, people are typically quite supportive. *(That's so great! You can do it!)* Yet when you actually begin adhering to a sustainable (dare I say enjoyable?) routine, and consequently lose weight in the process… they may not be so supportive anymore. You may encounter strong resistance from friends, family, and society in general. Once content and happy in your new lifestyle, you might now wonder if you are indeed doing something "annoying," "irksome," "unhealthy," or "bad" in your personal choices. Accusatory questions may fly:

> Some may attack your diet mentality:
> *Why are you so strict?*
> *Life's too short to not eat cake!*
> *Can't you loosen up?*
> *You're ruining the fun!*

> Others may zero in on the physical results of your diet:
> *You're losing too much weight!*
> *You're too skinny!*
> *You looked better when you weighed more!*

Then there are those who assume the "health" route:
That can't be healthy!
You're depriving yourself!
You need carbs!
Your metabolism is going to slow down!

I have been told all of these things and more. Given my *ever so slight* obsession with the science of health, the last ones distress me the most. All of this backlash can make you feel like an unreasonable Debbie Downer. Perhaps you *are* being too "intense" or "uptight," and *should* lighten up?

But wait! Before you proclaim *"to heck with it!"* and scarf down a piece of cake, donut, or even whole grain bread, take a moment to access the situation. Assuming you are indeed eating healthy (à la Paleo or intermittent fasting), why should what you do or do not eat affect others on such a personal level? Don't let other's insecurities or resentments intrude on your personal choices, *if such choices are healthy ones*. Know the reasoning and science of what you're doing, and if it is indeed healthy and sustainable, your lifestyle shall speak for itself! (If it's unhealthy and not sustainable, such will become evident and speak for itself.)

#REACTIONS TO INTERMITTENT FASTING

If you begin an intermittent fasting protocol, expect to hear *"Why aren't you eating?"* a lot. People tend to freak out when you don't eat. Like they just *freak out*. Once you have a few years of intermittent fasting under your belt, others more readily accept your habits. When I say I've been intermittent fasting daily for over 3 years, people often say *"Oh"* and stop asking questions. It's up to you whether you choose to "explain yourself," or simply ignore the subject. Arm yourself with knowledge about the science and benefits of fasting, and then choose wisely as to when to engage others on the subject, and when to let sleeping dogs lie.

Here are some of the various reactions to intermittent fasting you may encounter:

1. The Attacker
The Attacker becomes personally invested in a vendetta against you. I don't understand this response, as the Faster isn't intruding on the Attacker, but it happens. The Attacker

will berate you with insistences that your metabolism will shut down, you are not healthy, and you will die. It is best to just respond calmly with something like *"Ok,"* and then attempt to cease conversation or change the subject.

2. The Curious
The Curious is fascinated by your method of eating. He or she will ask you question after question. *(What do you eat? When do you eat? Aren't you starving? How do you do that? So like, you're not gonna eat any of this?)* The Curious is tolerable, assuming you are in a conversational mood.

3. The Sceptic
The Sceptic is highly doubtful of your logic, assuming the "questioning" mode of The Curious with a tinge of the hostility of the Attacker. The Sceptic will probably decide you are "crazy" at the end of said conversation, although they *might* dismiss the subject as a "personal choice." On rare occasions, the Sceptic may consider researching the topic a bit more.

4. The Fascinated
The Fascinated has just experienced a #mindblown moment, and is potentially open to joining the bandwagon. He or she also assumes the "questioning" mode of the Curious and Sceptic, yet with a warm and likely supportive enthusiasm. I love the Fascinated!

5. The Accepter
It is refreshing to encounter the Accepter. Libertarian in spirit, he or she simply says *"Ok,"* and shrugs when you delineate your eating plan. We need more Accepters in this world.

Chapter Twenty-Four

Supplements

Growing up, I always took a multivitamin, starting with the brightly colored, candy-esque "Flintstones" variety. We always ended up with a bottle full of orange vitamins, given the pink > purple > orange hierarchy. But supplements go far beyond the basic "vitamin," and my current personal supplement regime, ironically enough, excludes a multivitamin. Supplements may address nutritional deficits, improve body systems and functions, aid in combatting inflammation, or perhaps stimulate mental and/or physical activity. A Paleo lifestyle provides most of the "basic" vitamins, and you can supplement for specific needs from there.

I am listing supplements with which I have personal experience. One benefit of a clean diet is increased awareness of a supplement's effects (especially in the fasted state). I make a conscious effort to only change supplements one at a time, in order to ascertain changes from such. Supplements also affect everyone differently. Be sure to research and try things for yourself to see how you react.

A Note On Brands: Be careful in selecting brands. You want to make sure your supplements aren't loaded with unnecessary and potentially unhealthy/irritating fillers. (Magnesium stearate, for example, bothers me personally.) Good go-to brands, in my opinion, include *GAIA Herbs, Himalaya Herbal Healthcare, Jarrow Formulas, Life Extension, NOW Foods,* and *Source Naturals,* but always check individual labels for the specific ingredients! GAIA products in particular seem to feature extremely high quality herbs, with often liquid absorption and very minimal, if any, fillers. All specific product recommendations are my personal opinion. I am *not* affiliated with any of the companies or products.

ENERGY & ALERTNESS

While a good diet and sufficient sleep are the foundation for energy and alertness, I'm always looking for ways to enhance performance in a healthy manner, and without side effects. (10 cups of coffee or amphetamines are not the way to go here.)

CAFFEINE

Caffeine is the world's most widely used psychoactive drug (any chemical compound which affects the central nervous system). Readily available in coffee, tea, sodas, and energy drinks, caffeine is both lauded and condemned. I support regulated, smart caffeine use in the genesis of the day.

Caffeine boasts many positives. It provides a quick energy boost and stimulates the central nervous system and brain, increasing alertness. It raises the metabolism. Studies have shown caffeine can increase energy expenditure by 13%. It can also raise the thermic effect of food when taken with a meal (although I never do this personally). In exercise, caffeine encourages lipolysis and fat oxidation. It increases levels of free fatty acids in the bloodstream, aiding endurance and prolonging exhaustion. Caffeine can block adenosine, a chemical which increases muscle fatigue when exercising. In fact, caffeine has been shown to alleviate leg muscle pain during exercise. As for mood, caffeine stimulates the release of dopamine, the feel good "upper" chemical in the brain. Caffeine also features antioxidant properties and can protect cells from oxidative damage. Studies have linked caffeine consumption to decreased risk of diabetes, cancer, dementia, insulin resistance, and increased longevity.

That being said, caffeine is highly addictive. Its interplay with dopamine receptors creates re-enforcing effects, similar to the addictive mechanisms of cocaine and amphetamine. The brain also easily develops tolerance to caffeine, so that increasingly more of the substance is required in order to achieve the same positive effects. It is easy to increase intake past the beneficial amount and experience side effects. Overconsumption of caffeine can lead to jitters, heart palpitations, and insomnia. Caffeine withdrawal can be rather unpleasant, characterized by fatigue and headaches.

GINKGO BILOBA

An age old staple in traditional Chinese medicine, Ginkgo biloba has been shown to sharpen cognitive functioning by increasing blood flow to the brain and acting as an antioxidant, preventing free-radicals and oxidative stress. It supports membrane integrity and neurotransmitter activity. It may improve concentration while preventing memory loss, absentmindedness, confusion, tiredness, and feelings of depression. Gingko biloba has been used to treat neurodegenerative diseases such as Alzheimer's and dementia. Ginkgo biloba definitely seems to boost mental alertness for me personally. (Got some in me right now while writing this!) However, since studies disagree on Gingko's effect on the liver, I'm a bit wary. Some show a protective effect, while others link it to potential liver stress or damage. Go figure. The jury's still out.

GINSENG

Ginseng is one of the world's most widely taken herbal supplements. It is a natural energy booster which stimulates the central nervous system, supporting cognition and memory. As an adaptogen, ginseng helps regulate the stress response to promote homeostatsis (rather than merely serving as a stimulant, like caffeine). Clinical studies show ginseng may prevent fatigue, improve physical performance, support the immune system, and relieve stress.

The different types of ginseng include *Asian ginseng* (Panax), *American ginseng* (Panax quiquefolius), and *Siberian ginseng* (Eleutherococcus senticosus). In general, the Asian variety is the most stimulatory, and may raise blood pressure. The American version is "calmer," and thus better for stress relief and combatting adrenal fatigue. Siberian ginseng may aid environmental adaptations (like to temperature and altitude), combat stress and anxiety, and help with insomnia. Ginseng is often a staple in my morning supplementation. I seem to experience increased energy and alertness when using it.

L-TYROSINE

L-tyrosine is a nonessential amino acid involved in dopamine, epinephrine, and norepinephrine synthesis in the brain. It may help alleviate the effects of stress, while supporting mental alertness. Studies have shown it sustains cognitive function during physical stress. I stack L-tyrosine with caffeine for a more sustainable energy than from caffeine alone. It may be all in my head, but I truly feel that it "extends" the positive effects of caffeine, while minimizing any "crashing."

RHODIOLA ROSEA

Rhodiola rosea is an adaptogenic herb which supports a healthy stress response. Adaptogenic herbs work by regulating the body's stress response, rather than acting as mere stimulants (like caffeine, for example). Rhodiola has been shown to increase alertness and reduce fatigue in stressful situations, while minimizing negative effects. It also may support cognitive functioning, and be neuroprotective against toxins.

As an adaptogen, people react differently to rhodiola. If you're tired from a lack of cortisol (stress hormone), then rhodiola may seem stimulating to you. If you're burnt out from *too much* cortisol, however, then rhodiola may seem more calming. Either way, the herb works with your natural stress response to promote endurance. Rhodiola was a real winner for me personally. It definitely helped me combat high cortisol levels, and produced a constant, zen sort of energy.

SLEEP & STRESS

I strive for solid, sound sleep, but my overactive brain and reflections on life easily incite insomnia. It's a tricky business playing with herbal sleep supplements, since you want to achieve deep, restful sleep without feeling groggy the next morning. I recommend trying different supplements at different dosages to find what works best for you. (I'm still toying with the whole thing myself.) I do love teas formulated to support sleep, like Celestial Seasonings' "Sleepytime Extra" or Yogi's "Bedtime." Both feature valerian, in combination with other calming herbs, and definitely instigate feelings of well-being and sleepiness. Consuming the compounds in this liquid form also seems to aid their timely absorption. The following are natural sleep supplements which may benefit you.

CALCIUM/MAGNESIUM

You might not automatically associate it with sleep, but an adequately balanced calcium/magnesium ratio is *key* for sleep and relaxation. To start with the general health benefits, calcium is vital for bone mass and strength, especially for preventing osteoporosis. It also may be preventative against tumors and cancer, and supports good blood pressure. Magnesium is involved with all enzymes in the body using ATP for energy. It is vital for a healthy heart.

So how does calcium/magnesium relate to stress and sleep? Many people focus on getting adequate calcium, without paying attention to magnesium. The thing is, the two work synergistically, while being slightly "opposite" in nature, like two sides of a coin. Calcium is *excitatory* and instigates muscle contractions, while magnesium is *calming* and relaxes muscles. Excess calcium can actually deplete magnesium, resulting in an overexcited brain, lack of coherence, anxiety, and insomnia. I recommend ensuring a good calcium/magnesium ratio via a calcium/magnesium gel pill supplement, or with the "Natural Calm" drink, which is great for stress relief!

GABA

GABA is the primary inhibitory neurotransmitter in the brain. It may relieve anxiety and promote rest and relaxation. Anti-anxiety drugs known as benzodiazepines (like Xanax and Valium) actually act on GABA receptors.

KAVA KAVA

Kava kava comes from a plant grown in the South Pacific, with mild sedative and psychoactive effects. Kava is actually brewed in Polynesian islands as a calming, "feel-good" drink similar to alcohol. It may promote a calm mood and relieve both anxiety and insomnia. It has even been used as an alternative to antidepressants, without addictive side effects. Studies have linked kava to possible liver toxicity, so proceed with caution. Then again, these studies have been critiqued for including the actual poisonous part of the kava plant, rather than just the root. Yogi notably makes a "Kava Stress Relief" tea.

MELATONIN

Melatonin is a hormone secreted by the pineal gland which helps regulate the natural circadian rhythm and sleep cycle. It induces (rather than necessarily sustains) sleep, although it can improve sleep quality. It is non-addictive, with few, if any side effects, and does not encourage tolerance. It also seems to have no withdrawal effects. You can experiment with different dosages of melatonin, typically from 1-6 mg. Melatonin is best used in very small amounts to slowly adjust circadian rhythm, rather than high dosing.

L-THEANINE
L-theanine is an amino acid shown to reduce psychological and physiological stress responses, and to promote feelings of relaxation. You can stack it with caffeine to relieve caffeine's jitters in the morning, or take it at night to encourage a calmer mood.

VALERIAN
Herbal extracts of the flowering valerian plant promote anti-anxiety and sedation by acting on GABA receptors. The stuff can smell *absolutely terrible*, but it definitely has a nice effect. I've found it to be highly effective in brewed tea form, à la Yogi's "Bedtime" or Celestial Seasonings' "Sleepytime Extra."

HEALTHY GUT & DIGESTION
After understanding the foundational concept of Paleo, you probably "get" why a healthy gut is vital for overall health. Proper digestion is necessary to ensure that your body gets the nutrients it needs. It's where the fuel and building blocks of your life begin. No big deal. Bad digestion = bad news.

DANDELION
The dandelion herb can aid digestion, and also functions as a natural diuretic.

DIAMINE OXIDASE
Diamine oxidase is an enzyme required to break down histamines. If you have a specific food allergy, you may be able to supplement with diamine oxidase before the offending food to minimize negative reactions. When I was trying to pinpoint a personal food allergen, I found that supplementing with "Histame" or Swanson's "Daosin" (both containing diamine oxidase) severely minimized my allergic reactions.

L-GLUTAMINE

L-glutamine is an essential amino acid found throughout the body, but particularly in muscle. It aids in protein synthesis and helps prevent muscle breakdown. It is notably important for maintaining strength integrity of the intestinal track by preventing atrophy and permeability. Stress can reduce glutamine levels, so supplementation may be helpful. I started taking L-glutamine to support my digestive tract, but enjoyed the side benefit of enhanced muscle support and size.

HYDROCHLORIC ACID (HCL)

Hydrochloric Acid is a digestive acid produced in the stomach to break down food (primarily protein and fat). A multitude of factors can lead to decreased levels of HCL, particularly age and acute or chronic stress. Supplementing with HCL capsules before eating may reduce digestive problems if a lack of acid production is indeed the problem. The general recommendation is to start with the minimum dosage, then slowly increase each time you eat by one capsule. When you feel a "warm" sensation in your stomach, plateau at that number of capsules, before eventually titrating off. (Using HCL will stimulate your stomach to start producing more HCL of its own.)

Supplementing with HCL is perhaps more "serious" than most supplements, in that it will have a *very* definite effect one way or the other, so do your research and proceed with caution. However, its benefits can be truly amazing. HCL definitely worked for me when a period of stress impacted my stomach acid levels.

PROBIOTICS

The overuse of antibiotics today significantly reduces the healthy bacteria in our intestinal tract. Probiotics are *key* in replenishing these healthy bacteria that we need, such as lactobacillus acidophilus and bifidobacteria bifidum. (Such names!) Taking probiotics supports healthy digestion, and may alleviate problems such as diarrhea, constipation, gas, bloating, and IBS, as well as inflammatory conditions and other autoimmune ailments stemming from digestive issues. I personally like to try out new probiotic strands and brands, rather than sticking to just one, in order to hopefully replenish the strands my body needs specifically. Many people find great success with the soil-based probiotic "Prescript-Assist." You can also get probiotic benefits from fermented, unpasteurized foods such as sauerkraut, kimchi, miso, tempeh, and kefir.

ANTI-INFLAMMATORIES

An anti-inflammatory diet is *key* in supporting overall health. Chronic inflammation wreaks havoc in the body, leading to a myriad of health issues. While Paleo in general yields an anti-inflammatory diet, the following supplements may help reduce inflammation, while providing numerous other health benefits.

BLACK SEED OIL

"There is healing in Black Seed for all diseases except death," says Islamic tradition. Black seed oil was even found in King Tut's tomb, so apparently *he* thought it was pretty important. Black seed oil bears strong anti-inflammatory, antioxidant, antimicrobial, and antiviral properties. It may protect the kidneys, liver, and other cells in general from toxins. You can supplement with black seed oil in pill or oil form, and cook with it if you like the taste. (Most people don't, as it's slightly reminiscent of tea tree oil.)

CURCUMIN/ TURMERIC

Curcumin is the active ingredient in the Indian spice turmeric - a wonder plant with a myriad of powerful antioxidant, anti-inflammatory, antibacterial, and antiviral benefits. It also aids the liver, and may be preventative against cancer and cataract damage. In fact, studies indicate curcumin is as effective as cortisone for decreasing inflammation, yet without side effects. It scavenges reactive oxygen radicals in inflammation, and blocks pain neurotransmitters. If you have any sort of pain, ailment, skin condition, or gastrointestinal problem, turmeric or curcumin can probably help. You can take turmeric or curcumin specifically as a supplement, or cook with turmeric. (It's the yellow spice which flavors curries.) I recommend the later: turmeric is tasty!

GINGER

Ginger is an anti-inflammatory plant which particularly aids digestion and helps with nausea, motion sickness, and upset stomachs. It also strengthens intestinal membranes, and may reduce the risk of cancer. You can take ginger as a supplement, or cook with it in root or powder form. Ginger is literally my favorite spice EVER. I could eat it with every meal. Or plain. (Which I do.)

FISH OIL

Fish oil is high in anti-inflammatory Omega-3 fatty acids, one of the two essential fatty acids (EFAs) which *must* be consumed from food. The other EFA is Omega-6 (found in grains, nuts, and seeds), which is abundant in our modern diet and actually *inflammatory* in nature. A healthy Omega-6:3 ratio is 1:1, although today's common ratio is more like 16:1 - quite inflammatory! Consistent intake of Omega-3 via fish oil can help counter the detrimental effects of high Omega-6 consumption.

Omega-3s constitute cell membranes throughout the body. They are highly anti-inflammatory, supporting the immune system. They're protective of heart health, discouraging arrhythmia, ventricular enlargement, cardiovascular disease, and heart attacks. They lower triglyecerides, blood pressure, and "bad" LDL cholesterol. They support a good mood.

Fish Oil is specifically rich in the long-chain Omega-3 fatty acids *EPA* and *DHA*, naturally found only in seafood and algae. A majority of Omega-3's health benefits are thanks to EPA and DHA. The body can convert the short-chain Omega-3 *ALA* (found in vegetarian sources like flaxseed and walnuts) into EPA and DHA, but it's a highly inefficient conversion limited to 5% or less.

Studies on fish oil specifically (rather than Omega-3 in general) have shown it may prevent colon cancer, enhance cognitive and visual development function of children, reduce body fat mass, stimulate lipid oxidation, and help with depression. (Depressed patients tend to have low concentrations of DHA.) One study found that arthritis patients who replaced NSAIDs with fish oil experienced increased pain relief. Another study even suggested that 20 lives per 1,000 heart attacks could be saved with fish oil!

Supplementation with Omega-3s is a notably slow process, as you have to gradually change the fat ratio in the individual cells of the body. Favor consistent, long-term supplementation of "smaller" amounts of Omega-3s (while minimizing Omega-6 consumption), rather than short-term, intense Omega-3 supplementation. With fish oil, commitment is key!

FLAXSEED OIL

Flaxseed oil is a vegetarian option for getting anti-inflammatory Omega-3 fatty acids. See the "Fish Oil" section above for an elaboration on Omega-3's benefits. While flaxseed is quite high in the essential short-chain fatty acid *ALA*, it does not contain the long-chain *EPA* and *DHA*, the crème de la crème of the Omega-3 fatty acids. While the body can convert ALA into EPA and DHA, it is an inefficient process. As such, flaxseed oil should be considered a backup or supplementary route for getting adequate amounts of Omega-3s, with fatty fish and fish oil taking precedence.

JOINT SUPPORT

Age, stress, and degenerative diseases such as osteoarthritis (the most common type of arthritis affecting 27 million people in the US) can wear away the cartilage in joints like the hips, knees, and spine. Rather than seeking relief by merely masking the inflammation with NSAIDs (which may just exacerbate the problem in the end), it is much more effective to address the root cause by providing the building blocks of cartilage in the first place.

Many joint support supplements combine **GLUCOSAMINE SULFATE, CHONDROITIN SULFATE,** and **METHYLSULFONYLMETHANE (MSM).** Glucosamine is an amino sugar building block of cartilage, while chondroitin is a complex carb which ensures adequate hydration of cartilage. MSM is a sulfurous compound important for collagen synthesis, which plays a vital role in connective tissue. Using these supplements encourages joint repair while protecting against future damage, and can alleviate pain from arthritis, chronic back pain, muscle pain, tendinitis, carpal tunnel syndrome, temporomandibular joint syndrome (TMJ), post-traumatic pain, and degenerative joint diseases such as osteoarthritis. Since getting my wisdom teeth out, I've struggled with TMJ, and have found substantial relief with these supplements. "Osteo Biflex" is great, albeit pricey. I've also found success with the generic "Joint Support" supplement from *Trader Joe's*.

You can also support your joints and cartilage via food with **GELATIN** and **BONE BROTH**, formed from the protein collagen in animal connective tissue. (Who doesn't love jello-y treats?)

OTHER SUPPLEMENTS

ACTIVATED CHARCOAL

Activated charcoal is a superhero supplement for fighting toxins. Often used in water and air filters, activated charcoal is a processed form of carbon with a negatively charged, porous surface. It binds to positively charged chemicals and toxins, effectively ushering them through your digestive system. In fact, activated charcoal is so effective at toxin elimination, that it is often used in hospitals after poison overdoses. Forget toxin cleanses and such – activated charcoal may be the most genuinely effective anti-toxin agent available. You can take it internally to clear out toxins (it itself is nontoxic), or even brush your teeth with activated charcoal for teeth whitening! Activated charcoal should not be taken with medications or other supplements, however, as it may bind to them as well, inhibiting their absorption. Also, if there's one way to possibly prevent hangovers… activated charcoal may be it! If I'm ever feeling icky from accidentally consuming some nebulous food (or from a bit too much wine), activated charcoal can immediately clear my head and restore a positive mood.

B VITAMIN COMPLEX

B vitamins are necessary for a myriad of functions, primarily cell metabolism and energy. Because they are water soluble, B vitamins aren't stored in the body like fat soluble vitamins, so it's easy to become deficient. Consider a B complex to ensure you get all the different types of B vitamins you need!

> **B12:** This is the most complex and well known B vitamin "pitched" for energy levels. B12 is vital for energy metabolism in every single cell in the body. It is also involved in fatty acid and protein metabolism, as well as DNA synthesis. B12 deficiency can result in nervous tissue and brain damage, fatigue, bruising and bleeding, weight loss, digestive issues, shortness of breath, mania, psychosis, depression, irritability, as well as numerous other unpleasant conditions.
>
> **B1 (Thiamine):** Thiamine is a coenzyme involved in the metabolism of carbs and amino acids. Deficiencies can lead to loss of appetite, apathy, short-term memory loss, confusion, and irritability. Supplementation may improve well being, increase appetite, decrease fatigue, and alleviate menstrual cramps.
>
> **B2 (Riboflavin):** Originally known as Vitamin G, Riboflavin merges with proteins to form important enzymes. It may

prevent migraines, while a deficiency is linked to depression and schizophrenia.

B3 (Niacin): Niacin may delay the onset of diabetes, benefit cholesterol, prevent liver disease, aid arthritis, and treat schizophrenia.

B6 (Pyridoxine): Pyridoxine deficiency is linked to depression, carpal tunnel syndrome, and edema.

BIOTIN

Biotin is a B vitamin involved with the metabolism of fatty acids, primarily known for its support of healthy skin, hair, and nails. Biotin deficiencies can lead to hair loss, brittle nails, dermatitis, and skin rashes. Biotin is a staple in my routine, and I definitely notice a difference in my nail and hair strength when taking it.

CHOLINE

Choline is a water soluble B-like vitamin found primarily in eggs and meats. It supports healthy cell membranes, as well as brain and nerve function. It also aids in the metabolism of fats and "good" HDL cholesterol, protecting the liver from fat gain.

COQ10

Coenzyme Q10 is a nutrient found primarily in beef and eggs. It is an important part of the cell mitochondria, ensuring adequate energy production and regulation, endurance, and stamina. It also supports the heart, blood pressure, immune system, and may be preventative against diabetes and cancer. The amount of CoQ10 tends to decrease in the body with age, so supplementation can be helpful.

VITAMIN D

Vitamin D deficiency is prevalent in most populations. Vitamin D is a fat soluble vitamin (technically a "prohormone") important in the absorption and assimilation of nutrients. It is known as the "sunshine vitamin," since the body synthesizes it from sun exposure. (Although it is also found in fatty fish, with smaller amounts in mushrooms and egg yolks.) Vitamin D is particularly involved with calcium absorption and deposition, supporting bone health; deficiencies may lead to bone turnover, osteoporosis, and bone fractures. (If you increase calcium intake in your diet, you should similarly increase vitamin D intake.) Vitamin D is also involved with the immune system, insulin secretion, heart functioning, blood pressure regulation, and brain development. Levels of vitamin D in the body markedly decrease with age, so supplementation may be key, especially during winter months. Body fat gain and high cholesterol also negatively affect vitamin D levels. Definitely consider adding a vitamin D supplement (*vitamin D3* in particular) to your regime for optimal health!

EGCG
EGCG (Epigallocatechin gallate) is a catechin found in green tea. It is a potent antioxidant, with very strong anti-cancer properties. It also may inhibit fat gain and reduce fatigue. Sometimes I take EGCG in the morning, in the form of green tea pills.

MILK THISTLE EXTRACT (Silymarin)
Milk thistle, featuring the active component *silymarin*, supports a healthy liver, which is vital for the metabolism and assimilation of nutrients and elimination of toxins. Milk thistle extract helps repair damaged liver cells, encourages regeneration of liver cells and tissue, reduces inflammation, and protects the liver from future damage. It does this in part by scavenging free-radicals and preventing the oxidative degeneration of fats in the liver. It also alters the membranes of toxins to reduce their penetration. Milk thistle supplementation has shown great improvement in patients featuring liver damage from alcohol, and may also prevent cirrhosis.

OIL OF OREGANO
Oregano is a member of the mint family, and can serve as a natural antimicrobial, with potent antibacterial and antiviral properties. You can use oregano to support your immune system, fight off a cold, kill parasites, or combat small intestine bacterial overgrowth (SIBO). Oregano's active plant phytochemicals include thymol (a fungicide which can combat toxins) and carvacrol, which can combat bacterial infections. Oregano also supports respiratory health. Oregano is powerful stuff, best used in short bouts for specific purposes, rather than as a daily supplement.

PARSLEY
One of my slight obsessions is fresh breath. Parsley helps with

enzymatic deodorization, and may eliminate odors in the breath from food. I've found that it actually makes a difference if I take it before a garlicky meal (a personal demon).

RESVERATROL

Resveratrol is a polyphenol found in wine (particularly reds), and is linked to a myriad of health benefits. Resveratrol boasts anti-aging, antioxidant, and anti-inflammatory properties. It supports cardiovascular health, and may protect cells from degenerative diseases and cancer. Check out Chapter 21: *Alcohol and Diet* for more!

Conclusion

"Nothing will ever make me happy or satisfy me like my acting career. I will never be passionate about something like that."

    Such words were once my mantra. And yet the contents of this book stirred a happiness in me I never imagined. Perhaps it goes back to what we mean by being "happy." Deep down, I believe everything we do is motivated by that nebulous feeling of "happiness." We want contentment in our actions. To fulfill an innate sense of purpose. To do what we love. To be at peace with ourselves, our bodies, our decisions, our minds. *To feel good.*
    At first, weight loss was a path to a sort of metaphysical happiness. I thought if I was "skinny," I'd fulfill the aesthetic criteria for my dream job, and this would make me "happy." But in my quest for skinniness, I inadvertently stumbled into the health realm (which just so happens to be a very solid path to get there). Only then did I realize that a *chemical* happiness drives the *vague* happiness. Slenderness resulting from a body free of toxins and inflamed burdens can make you "happy" on a neurological level.
    This book focuses a lot on physical health and its corporeal benefits, with brief nods to the more cerebral experiences. Since I don't discuss it much in pages elsewhere, I'll touch on it here. The brain releases shots of the feel-good neurotransmitters *Dopamine, Serotonin, Oxytocin,* and *Endorphins* for activities and experiences it believes will sustain its existence. Whatever we pursue to "make us happy" involves the release of these chemicals. This system goes terribly wrong with addiction, when the body begins rewarding itself for dangerous habits, like discharging dopamine from highly palatable

junk foods. Such off-kilter neurotransmitters encourage a state of unattainable satisfaction, drowned in terrible side-effects like obesity and insulin resistance.

But on the flip side, a body free of stress, restriction, poisonous lifestyles, and excess, also fires these happy neurotransmitters, but in a *healthy* way. To get there, we've just got to attach these chemicals to good, natural things. How often do we visit the Tower of Babel, speaking in a foreign tongue to our body! "Calories" is *not* the terminology our body uses. Processed foods, chemicals, sugar, and grains (especially consumed 24/7), do *not* lead the body to successful livelihood, though they may beguile with dopamine or endorphin-fueled forlorn hope.

Maybe you can be thin and happy. Maybe you can have toned muscle without slaving away at a gym. Maybe you can eat for pleasure without addiction. Maybe you can have it all.

So many diet books are about losing weight. Getting to a certain scale number. Following a protocol for quick weight loss, because then you'll be "happy" in the vague sense. But it's not about that… not really. You just need to understand *why* the body does what it does. Then you can naturally lead it to a place you love. It'll go there on its own with the proper signals and circumstances. Leanness does not necessitate war. You *can* be satisfied and happy, both chemically and esoterically, with an effortlessly amazing body. All it takes is a changed perspective, embracing the *what* and the *when* to reach a wondrous place of satisfied sustainability.

THANKS (REALLY)

As the "stuff" of this book relates to my very real life, there are *quite* a few people I want to thank.

My family, for putting up with my half decade of crazy restaurant orders and grocery requests. And letting me eat their meat for dessert at restaurants. Specifically my Dad, for supporting me *always* and encouraging me to put passion into everything; my Mom, for caring so sincerely about my health; Danielle, for talking through anything and everything with me, and being ever so supportive of this book and all my freakout moments; Michael, for just being awesome. (He'll never read this.) To Carmen, for helping me shoot the most fabulous cover during our sensible Lizzie photoshoot. (So many outfits.) And for giving me so much feedback and insight on not only this project, but life in general. To my Paleo idol Robb Wolf, for fighting the good fight and changing my life, and who I feel like I know from listening to his podcast every day, and who actually retweeted my tweet that one time and MADE MY LIFE. To Andrew, for opening my eyes to the magical possibility of *actually* taking the proverbial pen to paper, and giving me the necessary tools when I was going to go the cheaper route. And for challenging me on stuff and never complaining when I decline lunch or order crazy things at dinner. To all my Facebook friends who specifically reached out to me about Paleo and Intermittent Fasting, and made me feel like maybe I actually wasn't crazy. (Thank you Stephanie for all of your amazing feedback and Oxford commas!) To Ben, for embarking on so many crazy diet adventures with me back in the day, and to Kara, for joining me in Paleoland. To Dallas, for always supporting my creative endeavors in this industry. To USC for teaching me how to research and write. (Although this section is a terrible example of it. #Streamofconsciousness.)

To Dopamine, Seratonin, Oxytocin, and Endorphins.

And of course, to God and life.

ABOUT THE AUTHOR

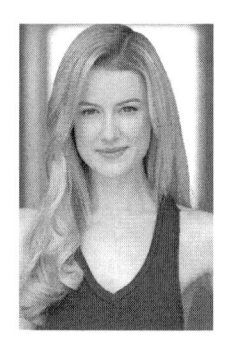

Born and raised in the South, Melanie Avalon left high school early to attend the early entrance program at the University of Southern California, during which time she interned for Jerry Bruckheimer, Julia Pistor, and Whitaker Entertainment at Walt Disney Studios. She received accolades for the highest GPA in the School of Theatre, the Louis Kerckhoff Prize for her paper "Charcot's Oppressive Hysteria: Vindicated Today?", and was a member of the Delta Kappa Alpha film fraternity and Phi Beta Kappa Honors Society. She graduated Summa Cum Laude, and is a member of Mensa International.

Melanie now works as an actress, writer, and audiobook recorder in Los Angeles. An "old soul," she's known for her vibrant, energetic, optimistic, magical nature. Her motto is, "Live vicariously through yourself!" She thanks Paleo and Intermittent Fasting for allowing her to maintain a slender, toned body for the entertainment industry, but without restriction, and awesome health to boot!

MelanieAvalon.com
PaleoActress.com
imdb.me/melanieavalon
twitter.com/melanieavalon
facebook.com/missmelanieavalon
youtube.com/c/melanieavalon

RESOURCES

A

Acheson, Kevin J., Gérard Gremaud, Isabelle Meirim, Franck Montigon, Yves Krebs, Laurent B. Fay, Louis-Jean Gay, Phillippe Schneiter, Charles Schindler, and Luc Tappy. "Metabolic Effects of Caffeine in Humans: Lipid Oxidation or Futile Cycling?" American Society for Clinical Nutrition 79.1 (2004): 40-46. Web.

Acheson, K. J., Y. Schutz, T. Bessard, K. Anantharman, J. P. Flatt, and E. Jéquier. "Glycogen Storage Capacity and De Novo Lipogenesis during Massive Carbohydrate Overfeeding in Man." American Journal of Clinical Nutrition 48.2 (1988): 240-47. Web.

Acheson, K.-H. J., B. Zahorska-Markiewicz, P. Pittet, K. Anantharaman, and E. Jéquier. "Caffeine and Coffee: Their Influence on Metabolic Rate and Substrate Utilization in Normal Weight and Obese Individuals." The American Journal of Clinical Nutrition 33.5 (n.d.): 989-97. Web.w

Agarwal, D. P. "Cardioprotective Effects Of Light-Moderate Consumption Of Alcohol: A Review Of Putative Mechanisms." Alcohol and Alcoholism 37.5 (2002): 409-15. Web.

Aggett, Peter J., Carlo Agostoni, Irene Axelsson, Christine A. Edwards, Olivier Goulet, Olle Hernell, Berthold Koletzko, Harry N. Lafeber, Jean-Léopold Micheli, Kim F. Michaelsen, Jacques Rigo, Hania Szajewska, and Lawrence T. Weaver. "Nondigestible Carbohydrates in the Diets of Infants and Young Children: A Commentary by the ESPGHAN Committee on Nutrition." Journal of Pediatric Gastroenterology and Nutrition 36.3 (2003): 329-37. Web.

Alberts, D. S., M. E. Martinez, D. J. Roe, J. M. Guillén-Rodríguez, J. R. Marshall, J. B. Van Leeuwen, M. E. Reid, C. Ritenbaugh, P. A. Vargas, A. B. Bhattacharyya, D. L. Earnest, and R. E. Sampliner. "Lack of Effect of a High-fiber Cereal Supplement on the Recurrence of Colorectal Adenomas. Phoenix Colon Cancer Prevention Physicians' Network." N Engl J Med 342.16 (2000): 1156-162. Web.

Ali, B. H., and Gerald Blunden. "Pharmacological and Toxicological Properties of Nigella Sativa." Phytotherapy Research 17.4 (2003): 299-305. Web.

Alirezaei, Mehrdad, Christopher C. Kemball, Claudia T. Flynn, Malcolm R. Wood, J. Lindsay Whitton, and William B. Kiosses. "Short-term Fasting Induces Profound Neuronal Autophagy." Autophagy 6.6 (2010): 702-10. Pubmed.gov. Web. 6 Sept. 2014.

Allen, Anthony K., G.paul Bolwell, David S. Brown, Christopher Sidebottom, and Antoni R. Slabas. "Potato Lectin: A Three-domain Glycoprotein with Novel Hydroxyproline-containing Sequences and Sequence Similarities to Wheat-germ Agglutinin." The International Journal of Biochemistry & Cell Biology 28.11 (1996):

1285-291. Web.

Amendola, Joseph, and Donald E. Lundberg. Understanding Baking. N.p.: Pan News, n.d. Print.

American College of Obstetricians and Gynecologists. "Obesity in Pregnancy." American College of Obstetricians and Gynecologists (2013): n. pag. Print. Committee Opinion No. 549. Obstet Gynecol 2013:121;213–7.

Anand, Preetha, Ajaikumar B. Kunnumakara, Chitra Sundaram, Kuzhuvelil B. Harikumar, Sheeja T. Tharakan, Oiki S. Lai, Bokyung Sung, and Bharat B. Aggarwal. "Cancer Is a Preventable Disease That Requires Major Lifestyle Changes." Pharmaceutical Research 25.9 (2008): 2097-116. Web.

Ancira, Kimberly, and Demand Media. "What Is the Difference Between Sucrose, Glucose & Fructose?" Healthyeating.sfgate.com. Hearst Communications, Inc., n.d. Web. 06 Sept. 2014. <http://healthyeating.sfgate.com/difference-between-sucrose-glucose-fructose-8704.html>.

Antonio, Jose, Corey A. Peacock, Anya Ellerbroek, Brandon Fromhoff, and Tobin Silver. "The Effects of Consuming a High Protein Diet (4.4 G/kg/d) on Body Composition in Resistance-trained Individuals." Journal of the International Society of Sports Nutrition 11.19 (2014): n. pag. Web.

Arima, Hisatomi, Yutaka Kiyohara, Isao Kato, Yumihiro Tanizaki, Michiaki Kubo, Hiromitsu Iwamoto, Keiichi Tanaka, Isao Abe, and Masatoshi Fujishima. "Alcohol Reduces Insulin–hypertension Relationship in a General Population The Hisayama Study." Journal of Clinical Epidemiology 55.9 (2002): 863-69. Jclinepi.com. Web. 6 Sept. 2014. Bartke, Andrew. "Insulin and Aging." Cell Cycle 7.21 (2008): 3338-343. Pubmed.gov. Web. 6 Sept. 2014.

"Aspartame Information Center." Aspartame.org. Calorie Control Council, n.d. Web. 07 Sept. 2014. <http://www.aspartame.org/>.

Avena, Nicole M., Pedro Rada, and Bartley G. Hoebel. "Evidence for Sugar Addiction: Behavioral and Neurochemical Effects of Intermittent, Excessive Sugar Intake." Neuroscience & Biobehavioral Reviews 32.1 (2008): 20-39. Web.

Azevedo, Fernanda Reis De, Dimas Ikeoka, and Bruno Caramelli. "Effects of Intermittent Fasting on Metabolism in Men." Revista Da Associação Médica Brasileira (English Edition) 59.2 (2013): 167-73. Web.

B

Baer, David J., Joseph T. Judd, Beverly A. Clevidence, and Russel P. Tracy. "Dietary Fatty Acids Affect Plasma Markers of Inflammation in Healthy Men Fed Controlled Diets: A Randomized Crossover Study." American Journal of Clinical Nutrition 79.6 (2004): 969-73. Web.

Barrett, Marilyn L., and Jay K. Udani. "A Proprietary Alpha-amylase Inhibitor from

White Bean (Phaseolus Vulgaris): A Review of Clinical Studies on Weight Loss and Glycemic Control." Nutrition Journal 10.1 (2011): 24. Web.

Barton, Debra L., Gamini S. Soori, Brent A. Bauer, Jeff A. Sloan, Patricia A. Johnson, Cesar Figueras, Steven Duane, Bassam Mattar, Heshan Liu, Pamela J. Atherton, Bradley Christensen, and Charles L. Loprinzi. "Pilot Study of Panax Quinquefolius (American Ginseng) to Improve Cancer-related Fatigue: A Randomized, Double-blind, Dose-finding Evaluation: NCCTG Trial N03CA." Supportive Care in Cancer 18.2 (2010): 179-87. Web.

Basu, Sanjay, Paula Yoffe, Nancy Hills, and Robert H. Lustig. "The Relationship of Sugar to Population-Level Diabetes Prevalence: An Econometric Analysis of Repeated Cross-Sectional Data." Ed. Bridget Wagner. PLoS ONE 8.2 (2013): E57873. Web.

Batchelor, A. J., and J.E. Compston. "Reduced Plasma Half-life of Radio-labelled 25-hydroxyvitamin D3 in Subjects Receiving a High Fiber Diet." British Journal of Nutrition 49 (1983): 213-16. Print.

Baumeister, Roy F., Ellen Bratslavsky, Mark Muraven, and Dianne M. Tice. "Ego Depletion: Is the Active Self a Limited Resource?" Journal of Personality and Social Psychology 74.5 (1998): 1252-265. Web.

Baumeister, Roy F., and Kathleen D. Vohs. "Self-Regulation, Ego Depletion, and Motivation." Social and Personality Psychology Compass 1 (2007): n. pag. Web.

Baumeister, Roy F., Matthew Gailliot, C. Nathan Dewall, and Megan Oaten. "Self-Regulation and Personality: How Interventions Increase Regulatory Success, and How Depletion Moderates the Effects of Traits on Behavior." Journal of Personality 74.6 (2006): 1773-802. Web.

Belko, Amy Z., and Teresa F. Barbieri. "Effect of Meal Size and Frequency on the Thermic Effect of Food." Nutrition Research 7.3 (1987): 237-42. Web.

Bellisle, France, Regina Mcdevitt, and Andrew M. Prentice. "Meal Frequency and Energy Balance." British Journal of Nutrition 77.S1 (1997): S57. Web.

Bergamini, Ettore. "Autophagy: A Cell Repair Mechanism That Retards Ageing and Age-associated Diseases and Can Be Intensified Pharmacologically." Molecular Aspects of Medicine 27.5-6 (2006): 403-10. Pubmed.gov. Web. 6 Sept. 2014.

Bieganski, T., J. Kusche, W. Lorenz, R. Hesterberg, C. Stahlknecht, and K. Feussner. "Distribution and Properties of Human Intestinal Diamine Oxidase and Its Relevance for the Histamine Catabolism." Biochimica Et Biophysica Acta (BBA) - General Subjects 756.2 (1983): 196-203. Web.

Biesiekierski, J. R., O. Rosella, R. Rose, K. Liels, J. S. Barrett, S. J. Shepherd, P. R. Gibson, and J. G. Muir. "Quantification of Fructans, Galacto-oligosacharides and Other Short-chain Carbohydrates in Processed Grains and Cereals." Journal of

Human Nutrition and Dietetics 24.2 (2011): 154-76. Web.

Bjarnason, Ingvar, and Ken Takeuchi. "Intestinal Permeability in the Pathogenesis of NSAID-induced Enteropathy." Journal of Gastroenterology 44.S19 (2009): 23-29. Web.

Blaak, Ellen. "Gender Differences in Fat Metabolism." Current Opinion in Clinical Nutrition and Metabolic Care 4.6 (2001): 499-502. Web.

Bocarsly, Miriam E., Elyse S. Powell, Nicole M. Avena, and Bartley G. Hoebel. "High-fructose Corn Syrup Causes Characteristics of Obesity in Rats: Increased Body Weight, Body Fat and Triglyceride Levels." Pharmacology Biochemistry and Behavior 97.1 (2010): 101-06. Web.

Bock, K. De, W. Derave, B. O. Eijnde, M. K. Hesselink, E. Koninckx, A. J. Rose, P. Schrauwen, A. Bonen, E. A. Richter, and P. Hespel. "Effect of Training in the Fasted State on Metabolic Responses during Exercise with Carbohydrate Intake." Journal of Applied Physiology 104.4 (2008): 1045-055. Web.

Boullata, Joseph I., and Angela M. Nace. "Safety Issues with Herbal Medicine: Common Herbal Medicines." Pharmacotherapy 20 (2000): 3. Print.

Bray, G. A., and B. M. Popkin. "Dietary Sugar and Body Weight: Have We Reached a Crisis in the Epidemic of Obesity and Diabetes?: Health Be Damned! Pour on the Sugar." Diabetes Care 37.4 (2014): 950-56. Web.

Bray, George A., Samara J. Nielsen, and Barry M. Popkin. "Consumption of High-fructose Corn Syrup in Beverages May Play a Role in the Epidemic of Obesity." American Journal of Clinical Nutrition 79.4 (2004): 537-43. Web.

Broadwell, R. D. "Transcytotic Pathway for Blood-Borne Protein through the Blood-Brain Barrier." Proceedings of the National Academy of Sciences 85.2 (1988): 632-36. Web.

Buman, Matthew P., Britton W. Brewer, Allen E. Cornelius, Judy L. Van Raalte, and Albert J. Petitpas. "Hitting the Wall in the Marathon: Phenomenological Characteristics and Associations with Expectancy, Gender, and Running History." Psychology of Sport and Exercise 9.2 (2008): 177-90. Web.

Burits, M., and F. Bucar. "Antioxidant Activity of Nigella Sativa Essential Oil." Phytotherapy Research 14.5 (2000): 323-28. Web.

Burr, M.l., J.f. Gilbert, R.m. Holliday, P.c. Elwood, A.m. Fehily, S. Rogers, P.m. Sweetnam, and N.m. Deadman. "Effects Of Changes In Fat, Fish, And Fibre Intakes On Death And Myocardial Reinfarction: Diet And Reinfarction Trial (Dart)." The Lancet 334.8666 (1989): 757-61. Web.

Businco, L., A. Cantani, M. A. Longhi, and P. G. Giampietro. "Anaphylactic Reactions to a Cow's Milk Whey Protein Hydrolysate (Alfa-Re, Nestle) in Infants with Cow's Milk Allergy." Annals of Allergy 62.4 (1989): 333-35. Web.

Butt, Masood Sadiq, and M. Tauseef Sultan. "Coffee and Its Consumption: Benefits and Risks." Critical Reviews in Food Science and Nutrition 51.4 (2011): 363-73. Web.

C

Cahill, G.f. "Starvation in Man." Clinics in Endocrinology and Metabolism 5.2 (1976): 397-415. Web.

"Carbohydrates." Http://www.hsph.harvard.edu. Harvard School of Public Health Nutrition Source, n.d. Web. 07 Sept. 2014. <http://www.hsph.harvard.edu/nutritionsource/carbohydrate-question/#sugar-alcohol>.

Carlson, Anton J., and Frederick Hoelzel. "Apparent Prolongation of the Life Span of Rats by Intermittent Fasting." The Journal of Nutrition 31.3 (1946): 363-75. The Journal of Nutrition. Web. 6 Sept. 2014.

Carlson, Michael G., Wanda L. Snead, and Peter J. Campbell. "Fuel and Energy Metabolism in Fasting Humans." American Journal of Clinical Nutrition 60.1 (1994): 29-36. ajcn.nutrition.org. Web. 6 Sept. 2014.

Cassidy, A., S. Bingham, and K. D. Setchell. "Biological Effects of a Diet of Soy Protein Rich in Isoflavones on the Menstrual Cycle of Premenopausal Women." The American Journal of Clinical Nutrition 60 (1994): 333-40. Web.

Cassimann, J. J. "Is Cancer a Hereditary or a Degenerative Disease?" Verh K Acad Geneeskd Belg 63.2 (2001): 137-52. Web.

Chowdhury, Golam MI, Lihong Jiang, Douglas L. Rothman, and Kevin L. Behar. "The Contribution of Ketone Bodies to Basal and Activity-dependent Neuronal Oxidation in Vivo." Journal of Cerebral Blood Flow & Metabolism 34 (2014): 1233-242. Web.

Church, Timothy S., Corby K. Martin, Angela M. Thompson, Conrad P. Earnest, Catherine R. Mikus, and Steven N. Blair. "Changes in Weight, Waist Circumference and Compensatory Responses with Different Doses of Exercise among Sedentary, Overweight Postmenopausal Women." Ed. Thorkild I. A. Sorensen. PLoS ONE 4.2 (2009): E4515. Web.

Claesson, Anna-Lena, Gunilla Holm, Åsa Ernersson, Torbjörn Lindström, and Fredrik H. Nystrom. "Two Weeks of Overfeeding with Candy, but Not Peanuts, Increases Insulin Levels and Body Weight." Scandinavian Journal of Clinical & Laboratory Investigation 69.5 (2009): 598-605. Web.

Clark, Nancy. Introduction. Nancy Clark's Sports Nutrition Guidebook. Champaign, IL: Human Kinetics, 2003. 143-52. Print.

Cohen, S., D. A. Tyrrell, M. A. Russell, M. J. Jarvis, and A. P. Smith. "Smoking, Alcohol Consumption, and Susceptibility to the Common Cold." American Journal of Public Health 83.9 (1993): 1277-283. Web.

Collier, R. "Intermittent Fasting: The Science of Going without." Canadian Medical Association Journal 185.9 (2013): E363-364. Web.

Cooper, Raymond, D. James Morré, and Dorothy M. Morré. "Medicinal Benefits of Green Tea: Part I. Review of Noncancer Health Benefits." The Journal of Alternative and Complementary Medicine 11.3 (2005): 521-28. Web.

Cooper, Raymond, D. James Morré, and Dorothy M. Morré. "Medicinal Benefits of Green Tea: Part II. Review of Anticancer Properties." The Journal of Alternative and Complementary Medicine 11.4 (2005): 639-52. Web.

Cordain, Loren. "Cereal Grains: Humanity's Double-Edged Sword." Evolutionary Aspects of Nutrition and Health: Diet, Exercise, Genetics and Chronic Disease. 84 (1999): 19-73. Web.

Cordain, Loren. "Modulation of Immune Function by Dietary Lectins in Rheumatoid Arthritis." Br J Nutr 83 (2000): 207-17. Web.

Corder, R., W. Mullen, N. Q. Khan, S. C. Marks, E. G. Wood, M. J. Carrier, and A. Crozier. "Oenology: Red Wine Procyanidins and Vascular Health." Nature 444.7119 (2006): 566. Web.

Cornell University. "Saponins." Cornell University Department of Animal Science. Cornell University, n.d. Web. 09 Sept. 2014.

Cox, L. S. "DNA Replication in Cell-free Extracts from Xenopus Eggs Is Prevented by Disrupting Nuclear Envelope Function." J Cell Sci. 101.1 (1992): 43-53. Web.

Coyle, Edward F. "The American Journal of Clinical Nutrition." American Journal of Clinical Nutrition 72.2 (2000): 512s-20s. Physical Activity As A Metabolic Stressor. Web. 08 Sept. 2014.

Criqui, M. "Does Diet or Alcohol Explain the French Paradox?" The Lancet 344.8939-8940 (1994): 1719-723. Sciencedirect.com. Web. 6 Sept. 2014.

Cummings, J. H., M. J. Hill, T. Jivraj, Helen Houston, W. J. Branch, and D. J.A. Jenkins. "The Effect of Meat Protein and Dietary Fiber on Colonic Function and Metabolism." American Journal of Clinical Nutrition 32 (1979): 2086-093. Web.

D

Dallosso, H. M., P. R. Murgatroyd, and W. P. James. "Feeding Frequency and Energy Balance in Adult Males." Human Nutrition. Clinical Nutrition 36C.1 (1982): 25-39. Web.

Darbinyan, V., A. Kteyan, A. Panossian, E. Gabrielian, G. Wikman, and H. Wagner. "Rhodiola Rosea in Stress Induced Fatigue — A Double Blind Cross-over Study of a Standardized Extract SHR-5 with a Repeated Low-dose Regimen on the Mental

Performance of Healthy Physicians during Night Duty." ScienceDirect.com. Elsevier, Oct. 2000. Web. 13 June 2015.

Das, Dipak K., Subhendu Mukherjee, and Diptarka Ray. "Erratum To: Resveratrol and Red Wine, Healthy Heart and Longevity." Heart Failure Reviews 16.4 (2011): 425-35. Link.springer.com. Web. 6 Sept. 2014.

Davidson, M. H., et al., "Safety and Endocrine Effects of 3-Acetyl-7-Oxo DHEA (7-Keto DHEA)," paper presented at Experimental Biology 98, April 19–22, 1998, San Francisco.

Davidson, Nancy K., and Peggy Moreland. "Why High Blood Sugar Is Bad." Mayoclinic.org. MayoClinic, 2 Mar. 2011. Web. 9 Sept. 2014.

Davies, M. J. "Effects of Moderate Alcohol Intake on Fasting Insulin and Glucose Concentrations and Insulin Sensitivity in Postmenopausal Women: A Randomized Controlled Trial." JAMA: The Journal of the American Medical Association 287.19 (2002): 2559-562. Jama.jamanetwork.com. Web. 6 Sept. 2014.

Davis, Ellen. "Cancer Cells Are Sugar Addicts: Using a Ketogenic Diet to Treat Cancer." Well Being Journal 22.5 (2013): 12-17. Web.

Dawson-Hughes, Bess, Robert P. Heaney, Michael F. Holick, Paul Lips, Pierre J. Meunier, and Reinhold Vieth. "Estimates of Optimal Vitamin D Status." Osteoporosis International 16.7 (2005): 713-16. Web.

Dean, Ward. "Beneficial Effects on Energy, Atherosclerosis and Aging." Nutrition Review (2013): n. pag. Http://nutritionreview.org. Web. 21 Sept. 2014. Web.

Deardorff, Julie. "Diabetes: Five Things You Didn't Know about Insulin Resistance." Chicagotribune.com. Tribune Newspapers, 31 Oct. 2012. Web. 07 Sept. 2014. <http://articles.chicagotribune.com/2012-10-31/health/sc-health-1031-diabetes-insulin-20121031_1_insulin-blood-sugar-diabetes-educator>.

Dees, Craig, James S. Foster, Shamila Ahamed, and Jay Wimalasena. "Dietary Estrogens Stimulate Human Breast Cells to Enter the Cell Cycle." Environmental Health Perspectives 105 (1997): 633. Web.

Deldicque, Louise, Katrien Bock, Michael Maris, Monique Ramaekers, Henri Nielens, Marc Francaux, and Peter Hespel. "Increased P70s6k Phosphorylation during Intake of a Protein–carbohydrate Drink following Resistance Exercise in the Fasted State." European Journal of Applied Physiology 108.4 (2010): 791-800. Pubmed.gov. Web. 6 Sept. 2014.

Department of Biochemistry and Division of Biomedical Sciences, University of California, Riverside, CA. "From Vitamin D to Hormone D: Fundamentals of the Vitamin D Endocrine System Essential for Good Health." The American Journal of Clinical Nutrition 88.2 (2008): 491S-99S. From Vitamin D to Hormone D: Fundamentals of the Vitamin D Endocrine System Essential for Good Health. American Journal of Clinical Nutrition. Web. 20 Oct. 2014.

"Diabetes: Differences Between Type 1 and 2-Topic Overview." WebMD.com. Healthwise, Incorporated, 26 Sept. 2012. Web. 04 Sept. 2014. http://www.webmd.com/diabetes/tc/diabetes-differences-between-type-1-and-2-topic-overview

Dohm, G. L., E. B. Tapscott, H. A. Barakat, and G. J. Kasperek. "Influence of Fasting on Glycogen Depletion in Rats during Exercise." Journal of Applied Physiology 55.3 (1983): 830-33. Web.

Dolapchieva, S. "Distribution of Concanavalin A and Wheat Germ Agglutinin Binding Sites in the Rat Peripheral Nerve Fibres Revealed by Lectin/glycoprotein-gold Histochemistry." The Histochemical Journal 28.1 (1996): 7-12. Web.

Dolfini, Ersilia, Leda Roncoroni, Luca Elli, Chiara Fumagalli, Roberto Colombo, Simona Ramponi, Fabio Forlani, and Maria T. Bardella. "Cytoskeleton Reorganization and Ultrastructural Damage Induced by Gliadin in a Three-dimensional in Vitro Model." World Journal of Gastroenterology 11.48 (2005): 7597-601. Web.

Drago, Sandro, Ramzi El Asmar, Mariarosaria Di Pierro, Maria Grazia Clemente, Amit Tripathi Anna Sapone, Manjusha Thakar, Giuseppe Iacono, Antonio Carroccio, Cinzia D'agate, Tarcisio Not, Lucia Zampini, Carlo Catassi, and Alessio Fasano. "Gliadin, Zonulin and Gut Permeability: Effects on Celiac and Non-celiac Intestinal Mucosa and Intestinal Cell Lines." Scandinavian Journal of Gastroenterology 41.4 (2006): 408-19. Web.

Duhigg, Charles. The Power of Habit: Why We Do What We Do In Life And Business. New York: Random House, 2012. 135-41. Print.

Dulloo, A. G., C. A. Geissler, T. Horton, A. Collins, and D. S. Miller. "Normal Caffeine Consumption: Influence on Thermogenesis and Daily Energy Expenditure in Lean and Postobese Human Volunteers." American Journal of Clinical Nutrition 49.1 (1989): 44-50. Web.

E

Eaton, S. Boyd, and Dorothy A. Nelson. "Calcium in Evolutionary Perspective." The Journal of Clinical Nutrition 1.54 (1991): 281S-87S. Web.

Eaton, S.boyd, Melvin Konner, and Marjorie Shostak. "Stone Agers in the Fast Lane: Chronic Degenerative Diseases in Evolutionary Perspective." The American Journal of Medicine 84.4 (1988): 739-49. Web.

Eaton, S. Boyd, and Melvin Konner. "Paleolithic Nutrition." New England Journal of Medicine 312.5 (1985): 283-89. Web.

Eberling, P., and V.a. Koivisto. "Physiological Importance of Dehydroepiandrosterone." The Lancet 343.8911 (1994): 1479-481. Web.

Evans, Suzette M., and Roland R. Griffiths. "Caffeine Tolerance and Choice in

Humans." Psychopharmacology 108.1-2 (1992): 51-59. Web.

EWG. "EWG's 2014 Shopper's Guide to Pesticides in Produce™." Ewg.org. Enviornmental Working Group, Apr. 2014. Web. 07 Sept. 2014. <http://www.ewg.org/foodnews/list.php>.

Ehrlich, Steven D. "Glutamine." University of Maryland Medical Center. VeriMed Healthcare Network, 7 May 2013. Web. 6 Sept. 2014.

Ehrlich, Steven D. "Milk Thistle." University of Maryland Medical Center. VeriMed Healthcare Network, 7 June 2013. Web. 6 Sept. 2014. <http://umm.edu/health/medical/altmed/herb/milk-thistle>.

Elia, M., C. Zed, G. Neale, and G. Livesey. "The Energy Cost of Triglyceride-fatty Acid Recycling in Nonobese Subjects after an Overnight Fast and Four Days of Starvation." Metabolism 36.3 (1987): 251-55. Sciencedirect.com. Web. 6 Sept. 2014.

Elliot, Sharon S., Nancy L. Keim, Judith S. Stern, Karen Teff, and Peter J. Havel. "Fructose, Weight Gain, and the Insulin Resistance Syndrome." American Journal of Clinical Nutrition 76.5 (2002): 911-22. Web.

Erdman, J. W. "Oilseed Phytates: Nutritional Implications." Journal of the American Oil Chemists' Society 56.8 (1979): 736-41. Web.

Erickson, Roger H., Johann Kim, Marvin H. Sleisenger, and Young S. Kim. "Effect of Lectins on the Activity of Brush Border Membrane-Bound Enzymes of Rat Small Intestine." Journal of Pediatric Gastroenterology and Nutrition 4.6 (1985): 984-91. Web.

Erlanson-Albertsson, Charlotte. "How Palatable Food Disrupts Appetite Regulation." Basic & Clinical Pharmacology & Toxicology 97.2 (2005): 61-73. Web.

F

Fälth-Magnusson, K., and K.-E. Magnusson. "Elevated Levels of Serum Antibodies to the Lectin Wheat Germ Agglutinin in Celiac Children Lend Support to the Gluten-lectin Theory of Celiac Disease." Pediatric Allergy and Immunology 6.2 (1995): 98-102. Web.

FAO. "Commodities by Country." Http://faostat.fao.org/site/339/default.aspx. Food and Agriculture Organization of the United Nations, n.d. Web.

Feinman, Richard D., and Eugene J. Fine. ""A Calorie Is a Calorie" Violates the Second Law of Thermodynamics." Nutrition Journal 3.9 (2004): 1-5. Web.

Fenwik, G. R., and R. K. Heaney. "Glucosinolates and Their Breakdown Products in Cruciferous Crops, Foods and Feedingstuffs." Food Chemistry 11.4 (1983): 249-71. Web.

Ferracioli-Oda, Eduardo, Ahmad Qawasmi, and Michael H. Bloch. "Meta-Analysis:

Melatonin for the Treatment of Primary Sleep Disorders." Ed. Andrej A. Romanovsky. PLoS ONE 8.5 (2013): E63773. Web.

Ferrieres, J. "The French Paradox: Lessons for Other Countries." Heart 90.1 (2004): 107-11. Web.

Finlaysona, G., E. Bryant, J. E. Blundella, and N. A. Kingb. "Acute Compensatory Eating following Exercise Is Associated with Implicit Hedonic Wanting for Food." Physiology & Behavior 97.1 (2009): 62-67. Web.

Foster, A., and J. Kemp. "Glutamate- and GABA-based CNS Therapeutics." Current Opinion in Pharmacology 6.1 (2006): 7-17. Web.

Franklin, A. L., I. L. Chaikoff, and S. R. Lerner. "The Influence of Goitrogenic Substances on the Conversion in Vitro of Inorganic Iodide to Thyroxine and Diiodotyrosine By Thyroid Tissue With Radioactive Iodine as Indicator." J. Biol. Chem. 153 (1944): 151-62. Web.

Francis, George, Zohar Kerem, Harinder P. S. Makkar, and Klaus Becker. "The Biological Action of Saponins in Animal Systems: A Review." British Journal of Nutrition 88.06 (2002): 587. Web.

Franks, Paul W., Soren Brage, Jian'An Luan, Ulf Ekelund, Mushtaquar Rahman, I. Sadaf Farooqi, Ian Halsall, Stephen O'Rahilly, and Nicholas J. Wareham. "Leptin Predicts a Worsening of the Features of the Metabolic Syndrome Independently of Obesity**." Obesity 13.8 (2005): 1476-484. Web.

Franz, M. J. "Protein: Metabolism and Effect on Blood Glucose Levels." The Diabetes Educator 23.6 (1997): 643-51. Web.

Freiberg, M. S., H. J. Cabral, T. C. Heeren, R. S. Vasan, and R. Curtis Ellison. "Alcohol Consumption and the Prevalence of the Metabolic Syndrome in the U.S.: A Cross-sectional Analysis of Data from the Third National Health and Nutrition Examination Survey." Diabetes Care 27.12 (2004): 2954-959. Care.diabetesjournals.org. Web. 6 Sept. 2014.

Fritz, P., H. V. Tuczek, J. Hoenes, A. Mischlinski, A. Grau, C. Hage, A. Koenig, and G. Wegner. "Use of Lectin-immunohistochemistry in Joint Diseases." Acta Histochem Suppl. 36 (1988): 277-83. Web.

Fu, J., H. Chen, D. N. Soroka, R. F. Warin, and S. Sang. "Cysteine-conjugated Metabolites of Ginger Components, Shogaols, Induce Apoptosis through Oxidative Stress-mediated P53 Pathway in Human Colon Cancer Cells." Journal of Agricultural and Food Chemistry 62.20 (2014): 4632-642. Europepmc.org. Web. 6 Sept. 2014.

Freed, D. L. J. "Do Dietary Lectins Cause Disease?" Bmj 318.7190 (1999): 1023-024. Web.

Freeman, J. M., E. P. G. Vining, D. J. Pillas, P. L. Pyzik, J. C. Casey, and L. A. M. T. Kelly. "The Efficacy of the Ketogenic Diet---1998: A Prospective Evaluation of

Intervention in 150 Children." Pediatrics 102.6 (1998): 1358-363. Web.

G

Garrett, Bridgette E., and Roland R. Griffiths. "The Role of Dopamine in the Behavioral Effects of Caffeine in Animals and Humans."

Gaziano, J.michael, Thomas A. Gaziano, Robert J. Glynn, Howard D. Sesso, Umed A. Ajani, Meir J. Stampfer, Joann E. Manson, Julie E. Buring, and Charles H. Hennekens. "Light-to-moderate Alcohol Consumption and Mortality in the Physicians' Health Study Enrollment Cohort." Journal of the American College of Cardiology 35.1 (2000): 96-105. Sciencedirect.com. Web. 6 Sept. 2014.

German, J. Bruce, and Rosemary L. Walzem. "The Health Benefits of Wine." Annual Review of Nutrition 20 (2000): 561-93. Sciencedirect.com. Web. 6 Sept. 2014.

Gibson, Peter R., and Susan J. Shepherd. "Evidence-based Dietary Management of Functional Gastrointestinal Symptoms: The FODMAP Approach." Journal of Gastroenterology and Hepatology 25.2 (2010): 252-58. Web.

Graf, Ernst, and John W. Eaton. "Suppression of Colonic Cancer by Dietary Phytic Acid." Nutrition and Cancer 19.1 (1993): 11-19. Web.

Graf, E., K. L. Empson, and J. W. Eaton. "Phytic Acid. A Natural Antioxidant." The Journal of Biological Chemistry 262 (1987): 11647-1650. Web.

Griffin, R. Morgan. "How Anti-Inflammatory Drugs Work." WebMD.com. WebMD, n.d. Web. 07 Sept. 2014.

Grob, P. M., and M. A. Bothwell. "Modification of Nerve Growth Factor Receptor Properties by Wheat Germ Agglutinin." J Biol Chem. 258.23 (1983): 14136-4143. Web.

Goodhart, Robert S., and Maurice E. Shils. Modern Nutrition in Health and Disease. 6th ed. Philadelphia: Lea and Febinger, 1980. 134-38. Print.

Gunnars, Kris. "How to Optimize Your Omega-6 to Omega-3 Ratio." AuthorityNutrition.com. Http://authoritynutrition.com/, n.d. Web. 21 Sept. 2014.

Guyton, Arthur C., and John E. Hall. Textbook of Medical Physiology. 11th ed. Philadelphia: Saunders, 2005. Print.

Guzmán, Manuel, and Cristina Blázquez. "Ketone Body Synthesis in the Brain: Possible Neuroprotective Effects." Prostaglandins, Leukotrienes and Essential Fatty Acids 70.3 (2004): 287-92. Web.

H

Hallberg, L., L. Rossander, and A. B. Skånberg. "Phytates and the Inhibitory Effect of Bran on Iron Absorption in Man." American Journal of Clinical Nutrition 45.5

(1987): 988-96. Web.

Halberg, N. "Effect of Intermittent Fasting and Refeeding on Insulin Action in Healthy Men." Journal of Applied Physiology 99.6 (2005): 2128-136. Web.

Halmos, Emma P., Victoria A. Power, Susan J. Shepherd, Peter R. Gibson, and Jane G. Muir. "A Diet Low in FODMAPs Reduces Symptoms of Irritable Bowel Syndrome." Gastroenterology 146.1 (2014): 67-75. Web.

Hamer, H., D. Jonkers, K. Venema, S. Vanhoutvin, F. J. Troost, and R. J. Broomer. "Review Article: The Role of Butyrate on Colonic Function." Alimentary Pharmacology & Therapeutics 27.2 (2008): 104-19. Wiley Online Library. John Wiley & Sons, Inc., 26 Oct. 2007. Web. 13 June 2015.

Hamid, Rabia, and Akbar Masood. "Dietary Lectins as Disease Causing Toxicants." Pakistan Journal of Nutrition 8.3 (2009): 293-303. Web.

Hartz, A. J., S. Bentler, R. Noyes, J. Hoehns, C. Logemann, S. Sinift, Y. Butani, W. Wang, K. Brake, M. Ernst, and H. Kautzman. "Randomized Controlled Trial of Siberian Ginseng for Chronic Fatigue." Psychological Medicine 34.1 (2004): 51-61. Web.

Harvard Health Publications. "Glycemic Index and Glycemic Load for 100+ Foods." Glycemic Index and Glycemic Load for 100+ Foods. Harvard University, n.d. Web. 11 Sept. 2014.

Harvard Medical School. "Why Not Flaxseed Oil?" Health.harvard.edu. President & Fellows of Harvard College, Nov. 2006. Web. 10 Sept. 2014.

Harvard School of Public Health. "Fats and Cholesterol: Out with the Bad, In with the Good." Hsph.harvard.edu. The President and Fellows of Harvard College, n.d. Web. 21 Sept. 2014.

Harvie, M. N., M. Pegington, M. P. Mattson, J. Frystyk, B. Dillon, G. Evans, J. Cuzick, S. A. Jebb, B. Martin, R. G. Cutler, T. G. Son, S. Maudsley, O. D. Carlson, J. M. Egan, A. Flyvbjerg, and A. Howell. "The Effects of Intermittent or Continuous Energy Restriction on Weight Loss and Metabolic Disease Risk Markers: A Randomized Trial in Young Overweight Women." International Journal of Obesity 35.5 (2010): 714-27. Pubmed.gov. Web. 6 Sept. 2014.

Harber, M. P., A. R. Konopka, B. Jemiolo, S. W. Trappe, T. A. Trappe, and P. T. Reidy. "Muscle Protein Synthesis and Gene Expression during Recovery from Aerobic Exercise in the Fasted and Fed States." AJP: Regulatory, Integrative and Comparative Physiology 299.5 (2010): R1254-1262. Pubmed.gov. Web. 6 Sept. 2014.

Hatori, Megum, Christopher Vollmers, Amir Zarrinpar, Luciano DiTacchio, Eric A. Bushong, Shubhroz Gill, Mathias Leblanc, Amandine Chaix, Matthew Joens, James A.J. Fitzpatrick, Mark H. Ellisman, and Satchidananda Panda. "Time-Restricted Feeding without Reducing Caloric Intake Prevents Metabolic Diseases in Mice Fed a

High-Fat Diet." Cell Metabolism 15.6 (2012): 848-60. Web.

Heilbronn, L. K. "Effect of 6-Month Calorie Restriction on Biomarkers of Longevity, Metabolic Adaptation, and Oxidative Stress in Overweight Individuals: A Randomized Controlled Trial." JAMA: The Journal of the American Medical Association 295.13 (2006): 1539-548. Web.

Higdon, Jane. "Essential Fatty Acids." Lpi.oregonstate.edu. Linus Pauling Institute, Dec. 2005. Web. 09 Sept. 2014.

Hill, Andrew J. "The Psychology of Food Craving: Symposium on 'Molecular Mechanisms and Psychology of Food Intake'." Proceedings of the Nutrition Society 66.2 (2007): 277-85. Journals.cambridge.org. 30 Apr. 2007. Web. 6 Sept. 2014.

Hojlund, Kurt, Mette Wildner-Christensen, Ole Eshoj, Christian Skjærbæk, Jens J. Holst, Ole Koldkjær, Dorte M. Jensen, and Henning Beck-Nielsen. "American Physiological SocietyAmerican Journal of Physiology - Endocrinology and Metabolism." The American Journal of Physiology - Endocrinology and Metabolism 280.1 (2001): n. pag. Web. 08 Sept. 2014.

Hokama, Akira. "Roles of Galectins in Inflammatory Bowel Disease." World Journal of Gastroenterology 14.33 (2008): 5133. Web.

Ho, K. Y., J. D. Veldhuis, M. L. Johnson, R. Furlanetto, W. S. Evans, K. G. Alberti, and M. O. Thorner. "Fasting Enhances Growth Hormone Secretion and Amplifies the Complex Rhythms of Growth Hormone Secretion in Man." Journal of Clinical Investigation 81.4 (1988): 968-75. Ncbi.nlm.nih.gov. Web. 6 Sept. 2014.

Honjoh, Steven, T. Yamamoto, M. Uno, and E. Nishida. "Signalling through RHEB-1 Mediates Intermittent Fasting-induced Longevity in C. Elegans." Nature 457 (2009): 726-30. Pubmed.gov. US National Library of Medicine National Institutes of Health, 14 Dec. 2008. Web. 6 Sept. 2014.

Horton, Jenn. "Agave: Calories, Nutrition Facts, and More." WebMD.com. WebMD, LLC., 22 July 2014. Web. 07 Sept. 2014. <http://www.webmd.com/diet/features/the-truth-about-agave>.

Horton, T. J., and J. O. Hill. "Prolonged Fasting Significantly Changes Nutrient Oxidation and Glucose Tolerance after a Normal Mixed Meal." Journal of Applied Physiology 90.1 (2001): 155-63. Web.

Hsieh, Ming-Hsiung, Paul Chan, Yuh-Mou Sue, Ju-Chi Liu, Toong Hua Liang, Tsuei-Yuen Huang, Brian Tomlinson, Moses Sing Sum Chow, Pai-Feng Kao, and Yi-Jen Chen. "Efficacy and Tolerability of Oral Stevioside in Patients with Mild Essential Hypertension: A Two-year, Randomized, Placebo-controlled Study." Clinical Therapeutics 25.11 (2003): 2797-808. Web.

Huebner, F.r., K.w. Lieberman, R.p. Rubino, and J.s. Wall. "Demonstration of High Opioid-like Activity in Isolated Peptides from Wheat Gluten Hydrolysates." Peptides

5.6 (1984): 1139-147. Web.

Hui, J., and Steve L. Taylor. "Inhibition of in Vivo Histamine Metabolism in Rats by Foodborne and Pharmacologic Inhibitors of Diamine Oxidase, Histamine N-methyltransferase, and Monoamine Oxidase." Toxicology and Applied Pharmacology 81.2 (1985): 241-49. Web.

I

Imir, T., and A. D. Bankhurst. "Inhibition of Natural Killer and Interleukin 2-activated NF Cell Cytotoxicity by Monosaccharides and Lectins." Mikrobiyol Bul 21 (1987): 245-50. Web.

Ishizuki, Y. "The Effects on the Thyroid Gland of Soybeans Administered Experimentally in Healthy Subjects." Nippon Naibunpi Gakkai Zasshi 767 (1991): 622-29. Web.

Ivanov, Anton, and Yuri Zilberter. "Critical State of Energy Metabolism in Brain Slices: The Principal Role of Oxygen Delivery and Energy Substrates in Shaping Neuronal Activity." Frontiers in Neuroenergetics 3 (2011): n. pag. Web.

Izumida, Yoshihiko, Naoya Yahagi, Yoshinori Takeuchi, Makiko Nishi, Akito Shikama, Ayako Takarada, Yukari Masuda, Midori Kubota, Takashi Matsuzaka, Yoshimi Nakagawa, Yoko Iizuka, Keiji Itaka, Kazunori Kataoka, Seiji Shioda, Akira Niijima, Tetsuya Yamada, Hideki Katagiri, Ryozo Nagai, Nobuhiro Yamada, Takashi Kadowaki, and Hitoshi Shimano. "Corrigendum: Glycogen Shortage during Fasting Triggers Liver–brain–adipose Neurocircuitry to Facilitate Fat Utilization." Nature Communications 4 (2013): n. pag. Web.

J

Jacobs, E. T., A. R. Giuliano, D. J. Roe, J. M. Guillén-Rodríguez, L. M. Hess, D. S. Alberts, and M. E. Martínez. "Intake of Supplemental and Total Fiber and Risk of Colorectal Adenoma Recurrence in the Wheat Bran Fiber Trial." Cancer Epidemiol Biomarkers Prev. 9 (2002): 906-14. Web.

Janick, Jules. "The Origins of Fruits, Fruit Growing, and Fruit Breeding." Hort.purdue.edu. Purdue University Department of Horticulture and Landscape Architecture, 2005. Web. 9 Sept. 2014.

Jankun, Jerzy, Steven H. Selman, and Rafai Swiercz. "Why Drinking Green Tea Could Prevent Cancer." Nature 3.387 (1997): 561. Print.

Jenkins, David J.A., Cyril W.C. Kendall, Livia S.A. Augustin, Silvia Franceschi, Maryam Hamidi, Augustine Marchie, Alexandra L. Jenkins, and Mette Axelsen. "Glycemic Index: Overview of Implications in Health and Disease." The American Journal of Clinical Nutrition 71.1 (2002): 266S-73S. Web.

Jenkins, D. J., T. M. Wolever,, R. H. Taylor, H. Barker, H. Fielden, J. M. Baldwin, A. C. Bowling, H. C. Newman, A. L. Jenkins, and D. V. Goff. "Glycemic Index of Foods:

A Physiological Basis for Carbohydrate Exchange." The American Society for Clinical Nutrition, Inc 34.3 (1981): 362-66. Ajcn.nutrition.org. The American Society for Clinical Nutrition, Inc. Web. 06 Sept. 2014.

Jenkinson, A., M. F. Franklin, K. Wahle, and G. G. Duthie. "Dietary Intakes of Polyunsaturated Fatty Acids and Indices of Oxidative Stress in Human Volunteers." European Journal of Clinical Nutrition 53.7 (1999): 523-28. Web.

Jensen, M. D., M. W. Haymond, J. E. Gerich, P. E. Cryer, and J. M. Miles. "Lipolysis during Fasting. Decreased Suppression by Insulin and Increased Stimulation by Epinephrine." Journal of Clinical Investigation 79.1 (1987): 207-13. Web.

Jensen, M. D., P. E. Cryer, C. M. Johnson, and M. J. Murray. "Effects of Epinephrine on Regional Free Fatty Acid and Energy Metabolism in Men and Women." The American Journal of Physiology 1st ser. 270.2 (1996): E259-264. Web.

Jéquier, Eric. "Alcohol Intake and Body Weight: A Paradox." American Journal of Clinical Nutrition 69.2 (1999): 173-74. Ajcn.nutrition.org. Web. 6 Sept. 2014.

Johnson, J.b., S. John, and D.r. Laub. "Pretreatment with Alternate Day Modified Fast Will Permit Higher Dose and Frequency of Cancer Chemotherapy and Better Cure Rates." Medical Hypotheses 72.4 (2009): 381-82. Pubmed.gov. Web. 6 Sept. 2014.

Johnson, Paul M. "Addiction-like Reward Dysfunction and Compulsive Eating in Obese Rats: Role for Dopamine D2 Receptors." National Neuroscience 13.5 (2010): 635-41. Web.

Johnson, Paul M., and Paul J. Kenny. "Dopamine D2 Receptors in Addiction-like Reward Dysfunction and Compulsive Eating in Obese Rats." Nature Neuroscience 13.5 (2010): 635-41. Web.

Jongsma, Maarten A., and Caroline Bolter. "The Adaptation of Insects to Plant Protease Inhibitors." Journal of Insect Physiology 43.10 (1997): 885-95. Web.

Juneja, L. "L-theanine—a Unique Amino Acid of Green Tea and Its Relaxation Effect in Humans." Trends in Food Science & Technology 10.6-7 (1999): 199-204. Web.

K

Kanarek, Robin. "Psychological Effects of Snacks and Altered Meal Frequency." British Journal of Nutrition 77.S1 (1997): S105. Web.

Keesey, Richard E., and Matt D. Hirvonen. "Body Weight Set-Points: Determination and Adjustment." American Society for Nutritional Services 127.9 (1997): 1875S-883S. Web.

Kennedy, David O., and Andrew B. Scholey. "Ginseng: Potential for the Enhancement of Cognitive Performance and Mood." Pharmacology Biochemistry and Behavior 75.3 (2003): 687-700. Web.

Kimura, Kenta, Makoto Ozeki, Lekh R. Juneja, and Hideki Ohira. "L-Theanine Reduces Psychological and Physiological Stress Responses." Biological Psychology 74.1 (2007): 39-45. Web.

Kim, Yong-Woon, and Philip J. Scarpace. "Repeated Fasting/refeeding Elevates Plasma Leptin without Increasing Fat Mass in Rats." Physiology & Behavior 78.3 (2003): 459-64. Web.

Kirkendall, Donald T., John B. Leiper, Zakia Bartagi, Jiri Dvorak, and Yacine Zerguini. "The Influence of Ramadan on Physical Performance Measures in Young Muslim Footballers." Journal of Sports Sciences 26.Sup3 (2008): S15-27. Pubmed.gov. Web. 6 Sept. 2014.

Kitano, N., T. Taminato, T. Ida, M. Seno, Y. Seino, S. Matsukura, S. Kuno, and H. Imura. "Detection of Antibodies against Wheat Germ Agglutinin Bound Glycoproteins on the Islet-cell Membrane." Diabetic Medicine 5.2 (1988): 139-44. Web.

Klaus, S., S. Pültz, C. Thöne-Reineke, and S. Wolfram. "Epigallocatechin Gallate Attenuates Diet-induced Obesity in Mice by Decreasing Energy Absorption and Increasing Fat Oxidation." International Journal of Obesity 29.6 (2005): 615-23. Web.

Klempel, Monica C., Surabhi Bhutani, Marian Fitzgibbon, Sally Freels, and Krista A. Varady. "Dietary and Physical Activity Adaptations to Alternate Day Modified Fasting: Implications for Optimal Weight Loss." Nutrition Journal 9.1 (2010): 35. Biomedcentral.com. Web. 6 Sept. 2014.

Knapik, J. J., C. N. Meredith, B. H. Jones, L. Suek, V. R. Young, and W. J. Evans. "Influence of Fasting on Carbohydrate and Fat Metabolism during Rest and Exercise in Men." Journal of Applied Physiology 64.5 (1998): 1923-929. Web.

Kokavec, Anna. "Is Decreased Appetite for Food a Physiological Consequence of Alcohol Consumption?" Appetite 51.2 (2008): 233-43. Sciencedirect.com. Web. 6 Sept. 2014.

Kobayaski, K., Y. Nagato, N. Aoi, L. R. Juneja, M. Kim, T. Yamamoto, and S. Sugimoto. "Effects of L-theanine on the Release of α-brain Waves in Human Volunteers." Journal of Japan Society for Bioscience, Biotechnology, and Agrochemistry 72.2 (1998): 153-57. Web.

Kolberg, J., and L. Sollid. "Lectin Activity of Gluten Identified as Wheat Germ Agglutinin." Biochemical and Biophysical Research Communications 130.2 (1985): 867-72. Web.

König, Bettina, Christine Rauer, Susann Rosenbaum, Corinna Brandsch, Klaus Eder, and Gabriele I. Stangl. "Fasting Upregulates PPARα Target Genes in Brain and

Influences Pituitary Hormone Expression in a PPARα Dependent Manner." PPAR Research 2009 (2009): 1-9. Web.

Kopp, P. "Resveratrol, a Phytoestrogen Found in Red Wine. A Possible Explanation for the Conundrum of the 'French Paradox'?" European Journal of Endocrinology 138.6 (1998): 619-20. Web.

Kovsan, Julia, Nava Bashan, Andrew S. Greenberg, and Assaf Rudich. "Potential Role of Autophagy in Modulation of Lipid Metabolism." American Journal of Physiology - Endocrinology and Metabolism 298.1 (2010): E1-E7. The-aps.org. Web. 6 Sept. 2014.

Kwon, J. Y., S. G. Seo, Y.-S. Heo, S. Yue, J.-X. Cheng, K. W. Lee, and K.-H. Kim. "Piceatannol, Natural Polyphenolic Stilbene, Inhibits Adipogenesis via Modulation of Mitotic Clonal Expansion and Insulin Receptor-dependent Insulin Signaling in Early Phase of Differentiation." Journal of Biological Chemistry 287.14 (2012): 11566-1578. Web.

L

Langner, S., E. Greifenberg, and J. Gruenwald. "Ginger: History and Use." Advances in Therapy 15.1 (1998): 25-44. Europepmc.org. Web. 6 Sept. 2014.

Lappalainen, R., P. O. Sjödén, T. Hursti, and V. Vesa. "Hunger/craving Responses and Reactivity to Food Stimuli during Fasting and Dieting." International Journal of Obesity 14.8 (n.d.): 679-88. Http://europepmc.org. Web. 6 Sept. 2014.

Laurin, Pia, Mats Wolving, and Karin Fälth-Magnusson. "Even Small Amounts of Gluten Cause Relapse in Children With Celiac Disease." Journal of Pediatric Gastroenterology and Nutrition 34.1 (2002): 26-30. Web.

Lemoine, Patrick, Tali Nir, Moshe Laudon, and Nava Zisapel. "Prolonged-release Melatonin Improves Sleep Quality and Morning Alertness in Insomnia Patients Aged 55 years and Older and Has No Withdrawal Effects." Journal of Sleep Research 16.4 (2007): 372-80. Web.

Letenneur, Luc. "Risk of Dementia and Alcohol and Wine Consumption: A Review of Recent Results." Biological Research 37.2 (2004): n. pag. Pubmed.com. Web. 6 Sept. 2014.

Levi, Boaz, and Moshe J. Werman. "Long-Term Fructose Consumption Accelerates Glycation and Several Age-Related Variables in Male Rats." Journal of Nutrition 128.9 (1998): 1442-449. Web.

Levine, James A. "The "NEAT Defect" in Human Obesity: The Role of Nonexercise Activity Thermogenesis." Endocrinology Update 2.1 (2007): 1-8. Web.

Lieber, Charles S. "Perspectives: Do Alcohol Calories Count." American Journal of Clinical Nutrition 54.6 (1991): 976-82. Http://ajcn.nutrition.org. Web. 6 Sept. 2014.

Lionetti, Elena, and Carlo Catassi. "New Clues in Celiac Disease Epidemiology, Pathogenesis, Clinical Manifestations, and Treatment." International Reviews of Immunology 30.4 (2011): 219-31. Web.

Lipton, R. I. "The Effect of Moderate Alcohol Use on the Relationship between Stress and Depression." American Journal of Public Health 84.12 (1994): 1913-917. Http://www.ncbi.nlm.nih.gov. Web. 6 Sept. 2014.

Liu, Luc, H. Gu, H. Liu, Y. Jiao, K. Li, Y. Zhao, L. An, and J. Yang. "Protective Effect of Resveratrol against IL-1β-induced Inflammatory Response on Human Osteoarthritic Chondrocytes Partly via the TLR4/MyD88/NF-κB Signaling Pathway: An "in Vitro Study." International Journal of Molecular Sciences 15.4 (2014): 6925-940. Pubmed.gov. Web. 6 Sept. 2014.

Liu, Simin, Walter C. Willett, Meis J. Stampfer, Frank B. Hu, Mary Franz, Laura Sampson, Charles H. Hennekens, and JoAnn E. Manson. "A Prospective Study of Dietary Glycemic Load, Carbohydrate Intake, and Risk of Coronary Heart Disease in US Women." American Journal of Clinical Nutrition 71.6 (2000): 1455-461. Web.

Liu, W.k., S.c.w. Sze, J.c.k. Ho, B.p.l. Liu, and M.c. Yu. "Wheat Germ Lectin Induces G2/M Arrest in Mouse L929 Fibroblasts." Journal of Cellular Biochemistry 91.6 (2004): 1159-173. Web.

Liuzzi, Grazia M., Maria P. Santacroce, Willy J. Peumans, Els J.m. Van Damme, B. Dicte Dubois, Ghislain Opdenakker, and Paolo Riccio. "Regulation of Gelatinases in Microglia and Astrocyte Cell Cultures by Plant Lectins." Glia 27.1 (1999): 53-61. Web.

Lopez-Garcia, Esther, Matthias B. Schulze, James B. Meigs, JoAnn E. Manson, Nader Rifai, Meir J. Stampfer, Walter C. Willett, and Frank B. Hu. "Consumption of Trans Fatty Acids Is Related to Plasma Biomarkers of Inflammation and Endothelial Dysfunction1." Journal of Nutrition 135.3 (2005): 562-66. Web.

Lorenzsonn, V., and W. A. Olsen. "In Vivo Responses of Rat Intestinal Epithelium to Intraluminal Dietary Lectins." Gastroenterology 82.1 (1982): 838-48. Web.

Lorgeril, M. De, S. Renaud, P. Salen, I. Monjaud, N. Mamelle, J.l Martin, J. Guidollet, P. Touboul, and J. Delaye. "Mediterranean Alpha-linolenic Acid-rich Diet in Secondary Prevention of Coronary Heart Disease." The Lancet 343.8911 (1994): 1454-459. Web.

Lowe, Michael R., and Allen S. Levine. "Eating Motives and the Controversy over Dieting: Eating Less Than Needed versus Less Than Wanted." Obesity 13.5 (2005): 797-806. Onlinelibrary.wiley.com. Web. 6 Sept. 2014.

Ludvigsson, J. F., S. M. Montgomery, A. Ekbom, L. Brandt, and F. Granath. "Small-Intestinal Histopathology and Mortality Risk in Celiac Disease." JAMA: The Journal of the American Medical Association 302.11 (2009): 1171-178. Web.

Lutas, Andrew, and Gary Yellen. "The Ketogenic Diet: Metabolic Influences on

Brain Excitability and Epilepsy." Trends in Neurosciences 36.1 (n.d.): 32-40. Web.

Lydiard, R. B. "He Role of GABA in Anxiety Disorders." The Journal of Clinical Psychiatry 64 (2003): 21-27. Web.

Ly, Kiet A., Peter Milgrom, and Marilynn Rothen. "Xylitol, Sweeteners, and Dental Caries." Pediatric Dentistry 28.2 (2006): 154-63. Web.

M

Maclaughlin, J., and M. F. Holick. "Aging Decreases the Capacity of Human Skin to Produce Vitamin D3." Journal of Clinical Investigation 76.4 (1985): 1536-538. Web.

Magnuson, B. A., G. A. Burdock, J. Doull, R. M. Kroes, G. M. Marsh, M. W. Pariza, P. S. Spencer, W. J. Waddell, R. Walker, and G. M. Williams. "Aspartame: A Safety Evaluation Based on Current Use Levels, Regulations, and Toxicological and Epidemiological Studies." Critical Reviews in Toxicology 37.8 (2007): 629-727. Web.

Mahadevan, S., and Y. Park. "Multifaceted Therapeutic Benefits of Ginkgo Biloba L.: Chemistry, Efficacy, Safety, and Uses." Journal of Food Science 73.1 (2008): R14-19. Web.

Mantovani, Alberto, Cecilia Garlanda, Andrea Doni, and Barbara Bottazzi. "Pentraxins in Innate Immunity: From C-Reactive Protein to the Long Pentraxin PTX3." Journal of Clinical Immunology 28.1 (2008): 1-13. Web.

Masiero, Eva, and Marco Sandri. "Autophagy Inhibition Induces Atrophy and Myopathy in Adult Skeletal Muscles." Autophagy 6.2 (2010): 307-09. Pubmed.gov. Web. 6 Sept. 2014.

Masiero, Eva, Lisa Agatea, Cristina Mammucari, Bert Blaauw, Emanuele Loro, Masaaki Komatsu, Daniel Metzger, Carlo Reggiani, Stefano Schiaffino, and Marco

Massey, Anna, and Andrew J. Hill. "Dieting and Food Craving. A Descriptive, Quasi-prospective Study." Appetite 58.3 (2012): 781-85. Europepmc.org. Web. 6 Sept. 2014.

Mattson, Mark P. "Energy Intake, Meal Frequencty, And Health: A Neurobiological Perspective." Annual Review of Nutrition 25.1 (2005): 237-60. Web.

Mattson, Mark P., Wenzhen Duan, and Zhihong Guo. "Meal Size and Frequency Affect Neuronal Plasticity and Vulnerability to Disease: Cellular and Molecular Mechanisms." Journal of Neurochemistry 84.3 (2003): 417-31. Onlinelibrary.wiley.com. Web. 6 Sept. 2014.

Matovinović, J., and V. Ramalingaswami. "Therapy and Prophylaxis of Endemic Goitre." Bulletin of the World Health Organization 18.1-2 (1958): 233-53. Web.

Mauriege, P., J. Galitzky, M. Berlan, and M. Lafontan. "Heterogeneous Distribution of Beta and Alpha-2 Adrenoceptor Binding Sites in Human Fat Cells from Various Fat Deposits: Functional Consequences." European Journal of Clinical Investigation

17.2 (1987): 156-65. Web.

Mayes, P. A. "Intermediary Metabolism of Fructose." American Journal of Clinical Nutrition 58 (n.d.): 754S-65S. Web.

Mayo Clinic Staff. "Goiter." Mayoclinic.org. Mayo Foundation for Medical Education and Research, 2 Jan. 2014. Web. 08 Sept. 2014.

Mayo Clinic Staff. "Trans Fat Is Double Trouble for Your Heart Health." Mayoclinic.org. Mayo Foundation for Medical Education and Research, 6 Aug. 2014. Web. 21 Sept. 2014.

McBroom, Patricia. "Monkey Diet Is Richer in Vitamins and Minerals than Human Diet, UC Berkeley Anthropologist Discovers." University of California Berkeley Press Release [Berkeley] 18 May 1999: n. pag. Print.

Mccarty, M.f. "Does Regular Ethanol Consumption Promote Insulin Sensitivity and Leanness by Stimulating AMP-activated Protein Kinase?" Medical Hypotheses 57.3 (2001): 405-07. Web.

Melnik, B. "Diet in Acne: Further Evidence for the Role of Nutrient Signalling in Acne Pathogenesis – A Commentary." Acta Dermato Venereologica 92.3 (2012): 228-31. Web.

Mezey, Esteban, and Louis A. Faillace. "Metabolic Impairment And Recovery Time In Acute Ethanol Intoxication." The Journal of Nervous and Mental Disease 153.6 (1971): 445-52. Web.

Miller, M. J. S., X.-J. Zhang, X. Gu, E. Tenore, and D. A. Clark. "Exaggerated Intestinal Histamine Release by Casein and Casein Hydrolysate but Not Whey Hydrolysate." Scandinavian Journal of Gastroenterology 26.4 (1991): 379-84.

Mishkind, M. "Immunocytochemical Localization of Wheat Germ Agglutinin in Wheat." The Journal of Cell Biology 92.3 (1982): 753-64. Web.

Mishkind, M. L., B. A. Palevitz, N. V. Raikhel, and K. Keegstra. "Localization of Wheat Germ Agglutinin--like Lectins in Various Species of the Gramineae." Science's STKE 220.4603 (1983): 1290-292. Web.

Miyake, Katsuya, Toru Tanaka, and Paul L. Mcneil. "Lectin-Based Food Poisoning: A New Mechanism of Protein Toxicity." Ed. Richard Steinhardt. PLoS ONE 2.8 (2007): E687. Web.

Moerman, Clara J., H. Bas De Mesquita, and Sytske Runia. "Dietary Sugar Intake in the Aetiology of Biliary Tract Cancer." International Journal of Epidemiology 22.2 (1993): 207-14. Web.

Mohanty, Priya, Wael Hamouda, Rajesh Garg, Ahmad Aljada, Husam Ghanim, and Paresh Dandona. "Glucose Challenge Stimulates Reactive Oxygen Species (ROS) Generation by Leucocytes." The Journal of Clinical Endocrinology & Metabolism

85.8 (2000): 2970-973. Web.

Momken, I., L. Stevens, A. Bergouignan, D. Desplanches, F. Rudwill, I. Chery, A. Zahariev, S. Zahn, T. P. Stein, J. L. Sebedio, E. Pujos-Guillot, M. Falempin, C. Simon, V. Coxam, T. Andrianjafiniony, G. Gauquelin-Koch, F. Picquet, and S. Blanc. "Resveratrol Prevents the Wasting Disorders of Mechanical Unloading by Acting as a Physical Exercise Mimetic in the Rat." The FASEB Journal 25.10 (2011): 3646-660. Web.

Montalto, Massimo, Ferruccio D'onofrio, Luca Santoro, Antonella Gallo, Antonio Gasbarrini, and Giovanni Gasbarrini. "Autoimmune Enteropathy in Children and Adults." Scandinavian Journal of Gatroenterology 44.9 (2009): 1029-036. Web.

Moore, Rusty. "Lose Body Fat By Eating Just One Meal Per Day? - Fitness Black Book." Fitness Black Book. N.p., 26 June 2007. Web. 07 Sept. 2014.

Motl, Robert W., Patrick J. O'connor, Leslie Tubandt, Tim Puetz, and Matthew R. Ely. "Effect of Caffeine on Leg Muscle Pain during Cycling Exercise among Females." Medicine & Science in Sports & Exercise 38.3 (2006): 598-604. Web.

Mozaffarian, Dariush, Tobias Pischon, Susan E. Hankinson, Nader Rifai, Kaumudi Joshipura, Walter C. Willett, and Eric B. Rimm. "Dietary Intake of Trans Fatty Acids and Systemic Inflammation in Women." American Journal of Clinical Nutrition 79.4 (2004): 606-12. Web.

Munch, Ryan, and Sheryl A. Barringer. "Deodorization of Garlic Breath Volatiles by Food and Food Components." Issue Journal of Food Science Journal of Food Science 79.4 (2014): C526-533. Web.

Murgatroyd, P. R., M. L. H. M. Van De Ven, G. R. Goldberg, and A. M. Prentice. "Alcohol and the Regulation of Energy Balance: Overnight Effects on Diet-induced Thermogenesis and Fuel Storage." British Journal of Nutrition 75.01 (1996): 33. Http://journals.cambridge.org. Web. 6 Sept. 2014.

Murphy, Michelle, and Julian G. Mercer. "Intermittent Feeding Schedules—Behavioural Consequences and Potential Clinical Significance." Nutrients 6.3 (2014): 985-1002. Web.

Murray, Frank. 100 Super Supplements for a Longer Life. Los Angeles, CA: Keats Pub., 2000. Print.

N

Nachbar, Martin S., and Joel D. Oppenheim. "Lectins in the United States Diet: A Survey of Lectins in Commonly Consumed Review of the Literature1'." The American Journal of Clinical Nutrition 33 (1980): 2338-345. Web.

"National Diabetes InformationClearinghouse (NDIC)." Insulin Resistance and Prediabetes. National Institute of Diabetes and Digestive and Kidney Diseases, National Institutes of Health., June 2014. Web. 07 Sept. 2014. <http://

diabetes.niddk.nih.gov/dm/pubs/insulinresistance>. NIH Publication No. 14–4893

National Toxicology Program. "Toxicology and Carcinogenesis Studies of Kava Kava Extract (CAS No. 9000-38-8) in F344/N Rats and B6C3F1 Mice (Gavage Studies)." Natl Toxicol Program Tech Rep Ser 571 (2012): 1-186. Pubmed.gov. Web. 6 Sept. 2014. <http://www.ncbi.nlm.nih.gov/pubmed/22441424>.

NCBI. "Sucrose." Pubchem.ncbi.nlm.nih.gov. N.p., n.d. Web. 11 Sept. 2014.

NCCAM. "Questions and Answers: NIH Glucosamine/Chondroitin Arthritis Intervention Trial Primary Study." Http://nccam.nih.gov. U.S. Department of Health & Human Services, May 2002. Web. 12 Sept. 2014.

Nejad, Mohammad, Maryam Karkhane, Abdolrazagh Marzban, Ehsan N. Mojarad, and Kamran Rostamicorresponding. "Gluten Related Disorders." Gastroenterol Hepatol Bed Bench 5.1 (2012): S1-S7. Web.

Norrelund, H., K. S. Nair, J. O. L. Jorgensen, J. S. Christiansen, and N. Moller. "The Protein-Retaining Effects of Growth Hormone During Fasting Involve Inhibition of Muscle-Protein Breakdown." Diabetes 50.1 (2001): 96-104. Web.

Nöthlings, Ute, Suzanne P. Murphy, Lynne R. Wilkens, Brian E. Henderson, and Laurence N. Kolonel. "Dietary Glycemic Load, Added Sugars, and Carbohydrates as Risk Factors for Pancreatic Cancer: The Multiethnic Cohort Study." American Journal of Clinical Nutrition 86.5 (2007): 1495-501. Web.

NYU Langone Medical Center. "Medium-Chain Triglycerides." Med.nyu.edu. EBSCO Publishing, Aug. 2011. Web. 10 Sept. 2014.

O

Oakenfull, David. "Soy Protein, Saponins and Plasma Cholesterol." The American Society for Nutritional Sciences 131.11 (2001): 2971. Web.

Ong, Z. Y., and B. S. Muhlhausler. "Maternal "junk-food" Feeding of Rat Dams Alters Food Choices and Development of the Mesolimbic Reward Pathway in the Offspring." The FASEB Journal 25.7 (2011): 2167-179. Web.

Opie, L. H., and S. Lecour. "The Red Wine Hypothesis: From Concepts to Protective Signalling Molecules." European Heart Journal 28.14 (2007): 1683-693. Web.

"Oregano: Uses, Side Effects, Interactions and Warnings - WebMD." Natural Medicines Comprehensive Database. Therapeutic Research Faculty, 2009. Web. 13 June 2015.

Osbourn, Anne. "Saponins and Plant Defence — a Soap Story." Trends in Plant Science 1.1 (1996): 4-9. Web.

Ouyang, Xiaosen, Pietro Cirillo, Yuri Sautin, Shannon Mccall, James L. Bruchette, Anna Mae Diehl, Richard J. Johnson, and Manal F. Abdelmalek. "Fructose

Consumption as a Risk Factor for Non-alcoholic Fatty Liver Disease." Journal of Hepatology 48.6 (2008): 993-99. Web.

Owen, O. E., A. P. Morgan, H. G. Kemp, J. M. Sullivan, M. G. Herrera, and G. F. Cahill. "Brain Metabolism during Fasting*." Journal of Clinical Investigation 46.10 (1967): 1589-595. Web.

P

Papadopoulou, K. "Compromised Disease Resistance in Saponin-deficient Plants." Proceedings of the National Academy of Sciences 96.22 (1999): 12923-2928. Web.

Parker, Hilary. "A Sweet Problem: Princeton Researchers Find That High-fructose Corn Syrup Prompts Considerably More Weight Gain." Princeton.edu. Trustees of Princeton University, 22 Mar. 2010. Web. 09 Sept. 2014.

Pohler, Holly. "Caffeine Intoxication and Addiction." The Journal for Nurse PractitPedersen, Merete, Soren Jacobsen, Mette Klarlund, Bo V. Pedersen, Allan Wiik, Jan Wohlfahrt,ioners 6.1 (2010): 49-52. Web

Patisaul, Heather B., and Wendy Jefferson. "The Pros and Cons of Phytoestrogens." Frontiers in Neuroendocrinology 31.4 (2010): 400-19. Web.

Pearce, Fred. "The Sterile Banana." Conservationmagazine.org. University of Washington, 26 Sept. 2008. Web. 09 Sept. 2014.

Pedersen, M., S. Jacobsen, M. Klarlund, B. V. Pedersen, A. Wiik, J. Wohlfahrt, and M. Frisch. "Environmental Risk Factors Differ between Rheumatoid Arthritis with and without Auto-antibodies against Cyclic Citrullinated Peptides." *Arthritis Res Ther.* 8.4 (2006): R133. Web.

Pellegrina, Chiara Dalla, Omar Perbellini, Maria Teresa Scupoli, Carlo Tomelleri, Chiara Zanetti, Gianni Zoccatelli, Marina Fusi, Angelo Peruffo, Corrado Rizzi, and Roberto Chignola. "Effects of Wheat Germ Agglutinin on Human Gastrointestinal Epithelium: Insights from an Experimental Model of Immune/epithelial Cell Interaction." Toxicology and Applied Pharmacology 237.2 (2009): 146-53. Web.

Perlmutter, David. Brain Maker: The Power Of Gut Microbes To Heal And Protect Your Brain -- For Life. N.p.: Little, Brown, 2015. Print.

Pomari, Elena, Bruno Stefanon, and Monica Colitti. "Effects of Two Different Rhodiola Rosea Extracts on Primary Human Visceral Adipocytes." MDPI.com. Molecules, May 2015. Web. 13 June 2015.

Proeyen, K., K. Bock, and P. Hespel. "Training in the Fasted State Facilitates Re-activation of EEF2 Activity during Recovery from Endurance Exercise." European Journal of Applied Physiology 111.7 (2011): 1297-305. Pubmed.gov. Web. 6 Sept. 2014.

Proeyen, K. Van, K. Szlufcik, H. Nielens, K. Pelgrim, L. Deldicque, M. Hesselink, P.

P. Van Veldhoven, and P. Hespel. "Training in the Fasted State Improves Glucose Tolerance during Fat-rich Diet." The Journal of Physiology 588.21 (2010): 4289-302. Web.

Proeyen, K. Van, K. Szlufcik, H. Nielens, M. Ramaekers, and P. Hespel. "Beneficial Metabolic Adaptations Due to Endurance Exercise Training in the Fasted State." Journal of Applied Physiology 110.1 (2011): 236-45. Pubmed.gov. Web. 6 Sept. 2014.

Pusztai, A. "Dietary Lectins Are Metabolic Signals for the Gut and Modulate Immune and Hormonal Functions." Eur J Clin Nutr 47 (1993): 691-99. Web.

Pusztai, A., S. W. B. Ewen, G. Grant, D. S. Brown, J. C. Stewart, W. J. Peumans, E. J. M. Van Damme, and S. Bardocz. "Antinutritive Effects of Wheat-germ Agglutinin and Other N-acetylglucosamine-specific Lectins." British Journal of Nutrition 70.01 (1993): 313. Web.

Q

R

Rada, P., N.m. Avena, and B.g. Hoebel. "Daily Bingeing on Sugar Repeatedly Releases Dopamine in the Accumbens Shell." Neuroscience 134.3 (2005): 737-44. Web.

Raffaghello, Lizzia, Valter Longo, Changhan Lee, Fernando M. Safdie, Min Wei, Federica Madia, and Giovanna Bianchi. "Starvation-dependent Differential Stress Resistance Protects Normal but Not Cancer Cells against High-dose Chemotherapy." Growth Hormone & IGF Research 105.24 (2008): 8215-220. Pnas.org. Web. 6 Sept. 2014.

Rapoport, Benjamin I. "Metabolic Factors Limiting Performance in Marathon Runners." Ed. Philip E. Bourne. PLoS Computational Biology 6.10 (2010): E1000960. Web.

Rayssiguier, Y., E. Gueux, W. Nowacki, E. Rock, and A. Mazur. "Igh Fructose Consumption Combined with Low Dietary Magnesium Intake May Increase the Incidence of the Metabolic Syndrome by Inducing Inflammation." Magnes Res 19.4 (2006): 237-43. Web.

Reddy, N. R., S. K. Sathe, and D. K. Salunkhe. "Phytates in Legumes and Cereals." Advances in Food Research 28 (1982): 1-82. Web.

Rheumatoid Arthritis with and without Auto-antibodies against Cyclic Citrullinated Peptides." Arthritis Research & Therapy 8 (2006): R133. Arthritis-research.com. Web. 6 Sept. 2014.

Rodin, Judith. "Insulin Levels, Hunger, and Food Intake: An Example of Feedback Loops in Body Weight Regulation." Health Psychology 4.1 (1985): 1-24. Web.

R, Oh, and D. L. Brown. "Vitamin B12 Deficiency." American Family Physician 67.5

(2003): 979-86. Web.

Richardson, Nicola J., Peter J. Rogers, Nicola A. Elliman, and Russell J. O'dell. "Mood and Performance Effects of Caffeine in Relation to Acute and Chronic Caffeine Deprivation." Pharmacology Biochemistry and Behavior 52.2 (1995): 313-20. Web.

Richelsen, B. "Increased Alpha 2- but Similar Beta-adrenergic Receptor Activities in Subcutaneous Gluteal Adipocytes from Females Compared with Males." Eur J Clin Invest. 16.4 (1996): 302-09. Web.

Rock, C. "Primary Dietary Prevention: Is the Fiber Story Over?" European Journal of Cancer Supplements 4.1 (2006): 29. Web.

Roitman, M. F. "Dopamine Operates as a Subsecond Modulator of Food Seeking." Journal of Neuroscience 24.6 (2004): 1265-271. Web.

Rossetti, L., A. Giaccari, and R. A. Defronzo. "Glucose Toxicity." Diabetes Care 13.6 (1990): 610-30. Web.

Roth, G. S. "Biomarkers of Caloric Restriction May Predict Longevity in Humans." Science 297.5582 (2002): 811. Web

Ryu, Sungpil, Sung-Keun Choi, Seung-Sam Joung, Heajung Suh, Youn-Soo Cha, Soochun Lee, and Kiwon Lim. "Caffeine as a Lipolytic Food Component Increases Endurance Performance in Rats and Athletes." Journal of Nutritional Science and Vitaminology 47.2 (2001): 139-46. Web.

S

"Saccharin." Beverageinstitute.org. Beverage Institute For Health & Wellness, May 2012. Web. 07 Sept. 2014. <http://beverageinstitute.org/us/article/saccharin/>.

Säemann, Marcus D., Georg A. Böhmig, Christoph H. Österreicher, Helmut Burtscher,, Ornella Parolini, Christos Diakos, Johannes Stöckl, Walter Hörl, and Gerhard J. Zlabinger. "Anti-inflammatory Effects of Sodium Butyrate on Human Monocytes: Potent Inhibition of IL-12 and Up-regulation of IL-10 Production." The FASEB Journal. Institute of Immunology and Department of Internal Medicine III,, Oct. 2000. Web. 13 June 2015.

Salema, Mohamed Labib, and Mohammad Sohrab Hossainb. "Protective Effect of Black Seed Oil from Nigella Sativa against Murine Cytomegalovirus Infection." International Journal of Immunopharmacology 22.9 (2000): 729-40. International Journal of Immunopharmacology. Web.

Sanchez, Albert, J. L. Reeser, H. S. Lau, P. Y. Yahiku, R. E. Willard, P. J. McMillan, S. Y. Cho, A. R. Magie, and U. D. Register. "Role of Sugars in Human Neutrophilic Phagocytosi." American Journal of Clinical Nutrition 26.11 (1973): 1180-184. Web.

Sanchez-Monge, R., L. Gomez, D. Barber, C. Lopez-Otin, A. Armentia, and G. Salcedo. "Wheat and Barley Allergens Associated with Baker's Asthma. Glycosylated

Subunits of the Alpha-amylase-inhibitor Family Have Enhanced IgE-binding Capacity." Biochemical Journal 281 (1992): 401-05. Web.

Sandell, Mari A., and Paul A.s. Breslin. "Variability in a Taste-receptor Gene Determines Whether We Taste Toxins in Food." Current Biology 16.18 (2006): R792-794. Web.

Sandri. "Autophagy Is Required to Maintain Muscle Mass." Cell Metabolism 10.6 (2009): 507-15. Pubmed.gov. Web. 6 Sept. 2014.

Sapone, Anna, Karen M. Lammers, Giuseppe Mazzarella, Irina Mikhailenko, Maria Carteni, Vincenzo Casolaro, and Alessio Fasano. "Differential Mucosal IL-17 Expression in Two Gliadin-Induced Disorders: Gluten Sensitivity and the Autoimmune Enteropathy Celiac Disease." International Archives of Allergy and Immunology 152.1 (2010): 75-80. Web.

Sapone, Anna, Karen M. Lammers, Vincenzo Casolaro, Marcella Cammarota, Maria Giuliano, Mario De Rosa, Rosita Stefanile, Giuseppe Mazzarella, Carlo Tolone, Maria Russo, Pasquale Esposito, Franca Ferraraccio, Maria Carteni, Gabriele Riegler, Laura De Magistris, and Alessio Fasano. "Divergence of Gut Permeability and Mucosal Immune Gene Expression in Two Gluten-associated Conditions: Celiac Disease and Gluten Sensitivity." BMC Medicine 9.1 (2011): 23. Web.

Sasano, H., M. Rojas, and S. G. Silverberg. "Analysis of Lectin Binding in Benign and Malignant Thyroid Nodules." Arch Pathol Lab Med. 113.2 (1989): 186-89. Web.

Savita, S. M., K. Sheela, Sharan Sunanda, A. G. Shankar, Parama Ramakrishna, and Srinivas Sakey. "Health Implications of Stevia Rebaudiana." Journal of Human Ecology 15.3 (2004): 191-94. Web.

Schairer, C. "Menopausal Estrogen and Estrogen-Progestin Replacement Therapy and Breast Cancer Risk." JAMA: The Journal of the American Medical Association 284.20 (2000): 485-91. Web.

Schibler, Ueli, Juergen Ripperger, and Steven A. Brown. "Peripheral Circadian Oscillators in Mammals: Time and Food." Journal of Biological Rhythms 18.3 (2003): 250-60. Web.

Schultz, Wolfram. "Predictive Reward Signal of Dopamine Neurons." Journal of Neurophysiology 80.1 (1998): 1-27. Web.

Science Signaling. "Why Excess Glucose Is Toxic." Science's STKE 2006.320 (2006): Tw40. Web.

Select Committee of Nutrition and Human Needs United States Senate. Dietary Goals for the United States. Washington D.C.: US Government Printing Office, 1977. Print.

Shamsuddin, Abulkalam M. "Inositol Phosphates Have Novel Anticancer Function."

The Journal of Nutrition (125): 725S-32S. Print.

Shirlow, M. J., and C. D. Mathers. "A Study of Caffeine Consumption and Symptoms: Indigestion, Palpitations, Tremor, Headache and Insomnia." International Journal of Epidemiology 14.2 (1985): 239-48. Web.

Sienkiewicz-Szłapka, E., B. Jarmołowska, S. Krawczuk, E. Kostyra, H. Kostyra, and M. Iwan. "Contents of Agonistic and Antagonistic Opioid Peptides in Different Cheese Varieties." International Dairy Journal 19.4 (2009): 258-63. Web.

Sigthorsson, G., J. Tibble, J. Hayllar, I. Menzies, A. Macpherson, R. Moots, D. Scott, M. J. Gumpel, and I. Bjarnason. "Intestinal Permeability and Inflammation in Patients on NSAIDs." Gut 43.4 (1998): 506-11. Web.

Siler, Scott Q., Richard A. Neese, and Marc K. Hellerstein. "De Novo Lipogenesis, Lipid Kinetics, and Whole-body Lipid Balances in Humans after Acute Alcohol Consumption." American Journal of Clinical Nutrition 70.5 (1999): 928-36. Ajcn.nutrition.org. Web. 6 Sept. 2014.

Simopoulos, A.p. "The Importance of the Ratio of Omega-6/omega-3 Essential Fatty Acids." Biomedicine & Pharmacotherapy 56.8 (2002): 365-79. Web.

Singh, Brahma N., Sharmila Shankar, and Rakesh K. Srivastava. "Green Tea Catechin, Epigallocatechin-3-gallate (EGCG): Mechanisms, Perspectives and Clinical Applications." Biochemical Pharmacology 82.12 (2011): 1807-1821. Web.

Siri-Tarino, P. W., Q. Sun, F. B. Hu, and R. M. Krauss. "Meta-analysis of Prospective Cohort Studies Evaluating the Association of Saturated Fat with Cardiovascular Disease." American Journal of Clinical Nutrition 91.3 (2010): 535-46. Web.

Soeters, M. R., P. B. Soeters, M. G. Schooneman, S. M. Houten, and J. A. Romijn. "Adaptive Reciprocity of Lipid and Glucose Metabolism in Human Short-term Starvation." AJP: Endocrinology and Metabolism 303.12 (2012): E1397-1407. Http://classic.ajpendo.physiology.org. Web. 6 Sept. 2014.

Sollid, L. M., J. Kolberg, H. Scott, J. Ek, O. Fausa, and P. Brandtzaeg. "Antibodies to Wheat Germ Agglutinin in Coeliac Disease." Clin Exp Immunol. 63.1 (1986): 95-100. Web.

Sonko, Bakary J., Andrew M. Prentice, Peter R. Murgatroyd, Gail R. Goldberg, Marlinde LHM Van De Vena, and William A. Coward. "Effect of Alcohol on Postmeal Fat Storage." American Journal of Clinical Nutrition 59.3 (1994): 619-25. Http://ajcn.nutrition.org. Web. 6 Sept. 2014.

Sonksen, P., and J. Sonksen. "Insulin: Understanding Its Action in Health and Disease." British Journal of Anaesthesia 85 (2000): 69-79. Oxford University Press Journals. Oxford University Press, 2000. Web. 06 Sept. 2014.

Stoll, Andrew. "Populations Maintaining Historic Omega-6 to Omega-3 Ratios (approximately 1 to 1) Are Protected from Many of the Scourges of the Modern

Age." The Omega-3 Connection. New York: Simon and Schuster, 2001. 43. Print.

Stowell, Sean R., Connie M. Arthur, Marcelo Dias-Baruffi, Lilian C. Rodrigues, Jean-Philippe Gourdine, Jamie Heimburg-Molinaro, Tongzhong Ju, Ross J. Molinaro, Carlos Rivera-Marrero, Baoyun Xia, David F. Smith, and Richard D. Cummings. "Innate Immune Lectins Kill Bacteria Expressing Blood Group Antigen." Nature Medicine 16.3 (2010): 295-301. Web.

Streppel, M. T., M. C. Ocke, H. C. Boshuizen, F. J. Kok, and D. Kromhout. "Long-term Wine Consumption Is Related to Cardiovascular Mortality and Life Expectancy Independently of Moderate Alcohol Intake: The Zutphen Study." Journal of Epidemiology & Community Health 63.7 (2009): 534-40. Http://jech.bmj.com. Web. 6 Sept. 2014.

"Sucralose." Beverageinstitute.org. Beverage Institute For Health & Wellness, May 2012. Web. 07 Sept. 2014. <http://beverageinstitute.org/us/article/saccharin/>.

Sudheer, Adluri R., and Venugopal P. Menon. "Antioxidant and Anti-inflammatory Properties of Curcumin." Advances in Experimental Medicine and Biology 595 (2007): 105-25. Springer Link. Web. 6 Sept. 2014.

Suez, Jotham, Tal Korem, David Zeevi, Gili Zilberman-Schapira,, Christoph A. Thaiss, Ori Maza, David Israeli, Niv Zmora, Shlomit Gilad, Adina Weinberger, Yael Kuperman, Alon Harmelin, Ilana Kolodkin-Gal, Hagit Shapiro, Zamir Halpern, Eran Segal, and Eran Elinav. "Artificial Sweeteners Induce Glucose Intolerance by Altering the Gut Microbiota." Nature 514 (2014): 181-86. Nature.com. Nature Publishing Group, 17 Sept. 2014. Web. 13 June 2015.

Suter, P. M., E. Jequier, and Y. Schutz. "Effect of Ethanol on Energy Expenditure." American Journal of Physiology - Endocrinology and Metabolism 2nd ser. 266.4 (1994): :R1204-R12. Print.

T

Tachibana, Hirofumi, Kiyoshi Koga, Yoshinori Fujimura, and Koji Yamada. "A Receptor for Green Tea Polyphenol EGCG." Nature Structural & Molecular Biology 11.4 (2004): 380-81. Web.

Tanaka, Masaaki, Yoshitake Baba, Yosky Kataoka, Noriaki Kinbara, Yuko M. Sagesaka, Takami Kakuda, and Yasuyoshi Watanabe. "Effects of (−)-epigallocatechin Gallate in Liver of an Animal Model of Combined (physical and Mental) Fatigue." Nutrition 24.6 (2008): 599-603. Web.

Tan, Kok-Yang, and Francis Seow-Choen. "Fiber and Colorectal Diseases: Separating Fact from Fiction." World J Gastroenterol 13.31 (2007): 4161-167. Web.

Taubes, Gary. Good Calories, Bad Calories: Fats, Carbs, and the Controversial Science of Diet and Health. New York: Anchor, 2008. Print.

Taylor, M. A., and J. S. Garrow. "Compared with Nibbling, Neither Gorging nor a

Morning Fast Affect Short-term Energy Balance in Obese Patients in a Chamber Calorimeter." International Journal of Obesity 25.4 (2001): 519-28. Web.

Teicholz, Nina. "The Questionable Link Between Saturated Fat and Heart Disease." Http://online.wsj.com. The Wall Street Journal, 6 May 2014. Web. 21 Sept. 2014.

Thurston, G., P. Baluk, A. Hirata, and D. M. McDonald. "Permeability-related Changes Revealed at Endothelial Cell Borders in Inflamed Venules by Lectin Binding." American Journal of Physiology: Heart and Circulatory Physiology 271.6 (1996): H2547-2562. Web

Thuy, Sabine, Ruth Ladurner, Valentina Volynets, Silvia Wagner, Stefan Strahl, Alfred Königsrainer, Klaus-Peter Maier, Stephan C. Bischoff, and Ina Bergheim. "Nonalcoholic Fatty Liver Disease in Humans Is Associated with Increased Plasma Endotoxin and Plasminogen Activator Inhibitor 1 Concentrations and with Fructose Intake." Journal of Nutrition 138.8 (2008): 1452-455. Web.

Torchon, Emmanuelle, Matthew Hulver, Ryan McMillan, and Brynn Voy. "Fasting Rapidly Increases Fatty Acid Oxidation in White Adipose Tissue." The FASEB Journal 28.1 (2014): 269.2. Web.

Torre, M., A. R. Rodriguez, and F. Saura-Calixto. "Effects of Dietary Fiber and Phytic Acid on Mineral Availability." Critical Reviews in Food Science and Nutrition 30.1 (1991): 1-22. Web.

Tremel, H., B. Kienle, L. S. Weilemann, P. Stehle, and P. Fürst. "Glutamine Dipeptide-supplemented Parenteral Nutrition Maintains Intestinal Function in the Critically Ill." Gastroenterology 107.6 (1994): 1595-601. Web.

Tsenkova, V. K., D. Carr, C, L. Coe, and C. D. Ryff. "Anger, Adiposity, and Glucose Control in Nondiabetic Adults: Findings from MIDUS II." Journal of Behavioral Medicine 37.1 (2014): 37-46. Web.

Turner, James E., Daniella Markovitch, James A. Betts, and Dylan Thompson. "Nonprescribed Physical Activity Energy Expenditure Is Maintained with Structured Exercise and Implicates a Compensatory Increase in Energy Intake." American Journal of Clinical Nutrition 92.5 (2010): 1009-016. American Journal of Clincial Nutrition. Web.

U

UK-Committee-on-Toxicity. "Phytoestrogens and Health, Committee on Toxicity of Chemicals in Food, Consumer Products and the Environment." (2003): London

USDA. "National Organic Program: Organic Standards." Ams.usda.gov. USDA, 4 Apr. 2014nation. Web. <http%3A%2F%2Fwww.ams.usda.gov%2FAMSv1.0%2FNOPOrganicStandards>.

V

Varady, K. A. "Intermittent versus Daily Calorie Restriction: Which Diet Regimen Is More Effective for Weight Loss?" Obesity Reviews 12.7 (2011): E593-601. Web.

Varady, Krista A., and Marc K. Hellerstein. "Alternate-day Fasting and Chronic Disease Prevention: A Review of Human and Animal Trials." American Society for Clinical Nutrition 86.1 (2007): 7-13. Web.

Varady, K. A., D. J. Roohk, B. K. McEvoy-Hein, B. D. Gaylinn, M. O. Thorner, and M. K. Hellerstein. "Modified Alternate-day Fasting Regimens Reduce Cell Proliferation Rates to a Similar Extent as Daily Calorie Restriction in Mice." FASEB Journal 22.6 (2008): 2090-6. Pubmed.gov. 9 Jan. 2008. Web. 6 Sept. 2014. FASEB J. 2008 Jun;22(6):2090-6. doi: 10.1096/fj.07-098178. Epub 2008 Jan 9.

Vega, Virginia L., Rafael De Cabo, and Antonio De Maio. "Age And Caloric Restriction Diets Are Confounding Factors That Modify The Response To Lipopolysaccharide By Peritoneal Macrophages In C57Bl/6 Mice." Shock 22.3 (2004): 248-53. Web.

Verboeket-van De Venne, W. P., K. R. Westerterp, and A. D. M. Kester. "Effect of the Pattern of Food Intake on Human Energy Metabolism." British Journal of Nutrition 70.01 (1993): 103. Pubmed.gov. Web. 6 Sept. 2014.

Vollmers, C., S. Gill, L. Ditacchio, S. R. Pulivarthy, H. D. Le, and S. Panda. "Time of Feeding and the Intrinsic Circadian Clock Drive Rhythms in Hepatic Gene Expression." Proceedings of the National Academy of Sciences 106.50 (2009): 21453-1458. Web.

Volkow, Nora D., and Roy A. Wise. "How Can Drug Addiction Help Us Understand Obesity?" Nature Neuroscience 8.5 (2005): 555-60. Web.

W

Wadden, T. A., G. D. Foster, K. A. Letizia, and J. L. Mullen. "Long-term Effects of Dieting on Resting Metabolic Rate in Obese Outpatients." JAMA: The Journal of the American Medical Association 264.6 (1990): 707-11. Web.

Wang, Zhirong, Jiangang Zou, Kejiang Cao, Tze-Chen Hsieh, Yuanzhu Huang, and Joseph M. Wu. "Dealcoholized Red Wine Containing Known Amounts of Resveratrol Suppresses Atherosclerosis in Hypercholesterolemic Rabbits without Affecting Plasma Lipid Levels." International Journal of Molecular Medicine 16.4 (2005): 533-40. Spandidos-publications.com. Web. 6 Sept. 2014.

Watzl, Bernhard, Christian Neudecker, Gertrud M. Hänsch, Gerhard Rechkemmer, and Beatrice L. Pool-Zobel. "Dietary Wheat Germ Agglutinin Modulates Ovalbumin-induced Immune Responses in Brown Norway Rats." British Journal of Nutrition 85.04 (2001): 483. Web.

Weinsier, R. L., G. R. Hunter, P. A. Zuckerman, D. T. Redden, B. E. Darnell, D. E. Larson, B. R. Newcomer, and M. I. Goran. "Energy Expenditure and Free-living Physical Activity in Black and White Women: Comparison before and after Weight

Loss." American Journal of Clinical Nutrition 71.5 (2000): 1138-146. Web.

Westman, Eric C. "Is Dietary Carbohydrate Essential for Human Nutrition?" American Society for Clinical Nutrition 75.5 (2002): 951-53. Web.

Westman, Eric C., Richard D. Feinman, John C. Mavropoulos, Mary C. Vernon, Jeff S. Volek, James A. Wortman, William S. Yancy, and Stephen D. Phinney. "Low-carbohydrate Nutrition and Metabolism." American Journal of Clinical Nutrition 86.2 (2007): 276-84. Web.

"What You Eat Can Fuel or Cool Inflammation, a Key Driver of Heart Disease, Diabetes, and Other Chronic Conditions." What You Eat Can Fuel or Cool Inflammation, a Key Driver of Heart Disease, Diabetes, and Other Chronic Conditions. Harvard Medical School, Feb. 2007. Web. 07 Sept. 2014.

Wilmore, Douglas W. "Catecholamines: Mediator of the Hypermetabolic Response to Thermal Injury." Annals of Surgery 180.4 (1974): 653-68. Web.

Wolf, Robb, and David Perlmutter. "The Paleo Solution Podcast: Ep. 200." Audio blog post. Http://robbwolf.com. N.p., 17 Sept. 2013. Web. 11 Sept. 2014.

Wolf, Robb. The Paleo Solution: The Original Human Diet. Las Vegas: Victory Belt, 2010. Print.

Woznicki, Katrina. "How Red Wine Helps the Heart." WebMD.com. WebMD, 21 June 2010. Web. 06 Sept. 2014.

X

Xu, Xiangru, Mohamed R. Mughal, F. Scott Hall, Maria T. G. Perona, Paul J. Pistell, Justin D. Lathia, Srinivasulu Chigurupati, Kevin G. Becker, Bruce Ladenheim, Laura E. Niklason, George R. Uhl, Jean Lud Cadet, and Mark P. Mattson. "Dietary Restriction Mitigates Cocaine-induced Alterations of Olfactory Bulb Cellular Plasticity and Gene Expression, and Behavior." Journal of Neurochemistry 114.1 (2010): 323-34. Pubmed.gov. Web. 6 Sept. 2014.

Y

Yancy, W.s., M.k. Olsen, J.r. Guyton, R.p. Bakst, and E.c. Westman. "A Low-carbohydrate, Ketogenic Diet versus a Low-fat Diet to Treat Obesity and Hyperlipidemia." ACC Current Journal Review 13.8 (2004): 18-19. Web.

Yeh, T. C., C. P. Liu, W. H. Cheng, B. R. Chen, P. J. Lu, P. W. Cheng, W. Y. Ho., G. C. Sun, J. C. Liou, and C. J. Tseng. "Caffeine Intake Improves Fructose-induced Hypertension and Insulin Resistance by Enhancing Central Insulin Signaling." Hypertension 63.3 (2014): 535-41. Web.

Yeomans, Martin R. "Alcohol, Appetite and Energy Balance: Is Alcohol Intake a Risk Factor for Obesity?" Physiology & Behavior 100.1 (2010): 82-89. Sciencedirect.com.

Web. 6 Sept. 2014.

Yoon, J. Cliff, Pere Puigserver, Guoxun Chen, Jerry Donovan, Zhidan Wu, James Rhee, Guillaume Adelmant, John Stafford, Ronald Kahn, Daryl K. Granner, Christopher B. Newgard, and Bruce M. Spiegelman. "Control of Hepatic Gluconeogenesis through the Transcriptional Coactivator PGC-1." Nature 413 (2001): 131-38. Web.

Yoshida, M., N. M. McKeown, G. Rogers, J. B. Meigs, E. Saltzman, R. D'Agostino, and P. F. Jacques. "Surrogate Markers of Insulin Resistance Are Associated with Consumption of Sugar-sweetened Drinks and Fruit Juice in Middle and Older-aged Adults." Journal of Nutrition 137.9 (2007): 2121-127. Web.

Youdim, Kuresh A., and James A. Joseph. "A Possible Emerging Role of Phytochemicals in Improving Age-related Neurological Dysfunctions: A Multiplicity of Effects." Free Radical Biology and Medicine 30.6 (2001): 583-94. Web.

Young, Simon N. "L-Tyrosine to Alleviate the Effects of Stress?" Journal of Psychiatry & Neuroscience 32.3 (2007): 224. Web.

Z

Zauner, C., B. Schneeweiss, A, Kranz, C. Madi, K. Ratheiser, L. Kramer, E. Roth, B. Schneider, and K. :enz. "Resting Energy Expenditure in Short-term Starvation Is Increased as a Result of an Increase in Serum Norepinephrine." American Journal of Clinical Nutrition 71.8 (2000): 1151-155. Web.

Zelman, Kathleen M. "The Benefits of Fiber: For Your Heart, Weight, and Energy." WebMD.com. WebMD, LLC., n.d. Web. 07 Sept. 2014. <http://www.webmd.com/diet/fiber-health-benefits-11/insoluble-soluble-fiber>.

Ziegler, T. R., K. Benfell, R. J. Smith, L. S. Young, E. Brown, E. Ferrari-Baliviera, D. K. Lowe, and D. W. Wilmore. "Safety and Metabolic Effects of L-Glutamine Administration in Humans." Journal of Parenteral and Enteral Nutrition 14.4 Suppl (1990): 137S-46S. Web.

Zioudrou, Christine, Richard A. Streaty, and Werner A. Klee. "Opioid Peptides Derived from Food Proteins." The Journal of Biological Chemistry 254.7 (1979): 2446-449. Web.

Made in the USA
Middletown, DE
20 December 2015